SEXUAL ASSAULT IN THE MILITARY

Military Life

Military Life is a series of books for service members and their families who must deal with the significant yet often overlooked difficulties unique to life in the military. Each of the titles in the series is a comprehensive presentation of the problems that arise, solutions to these problems, and resources that are of much further help. The authors of these books—who are themselves military members and experienced writers—have personally faced these challenging situations, and understand the many complications that accompany them. This is the first stop for members of the military and their loved ones in search of information on navigating the complex world of military life.

1. *The Military Marriage Manual: Tactics for Successful Relationships* by Janelle Hill, Cheryl Lawhorne, and Don Philpott (2010).
2. *Combat-Related Traumatic Brain Injury and PTSD: A Resource and Recovery Guide* by Cheryl Lawhorne and Don Philpott (2010).
3. *Special Needs Families in the Military: A Resource Guide* by Janelle Hill and Don Philpott (2010).
4. *Sexual Assault in the Military: A Guide for Victims and Families* by Cheryl Lawhorne-Scott, Don Philpott, and Jeff Scott

SEXUAL ASSAULT IN THE MILITARY

A Guide for Victims and Families

CHERYL LAWHORNE SCOTT, DON PHILPOTT,
AND LtCol. JEFF SCOTT

ROWMAN & LITTLEFIELD
Lanham • Boulder • New York • Toronto • Plymouth, UK

Published by Rowman & Littlefield
4501 Forbes Boulevard, Suite 200, Lanham, Maryland 20706
www.rowman.com

10 Thornbury Road, Plymouth PL6 7PP, United Kingdom

British Library Cataloguing in Publication Information Available

Library of Congress Cataloging-in-Publication Data

Lawhorne Scott, Cheryl, 1968–
  Sexual assault in the military : a guide for victims and families / Cheryl
Lawhorne Scott, Don Philpott, and Jeff Scott.
    pages cm. — (Military life)
  Includes bibliographical references and index.
  ISBN 978-1-4422-2750-7 (cloth : alk. paper)—ISBN 978-1-4422-2751-4
(electronic)
  1. Sexual harassment in the military—United States. 2. Sexual abuse victims—
Services for—United States. 3. Rape—United States—Prevention. 4. Sexual
harassment in the military—United States—Prevention. 5. Women soldiers—
Crimes against—United States. 6. Soldiers—Crimes against—United States.
7. United States—Armed Forces—Women—Crimes against. I. Philpott, Don,
1946– II. Scott, Jeff, 1969– III. Title.
  UB418.W65L347 2013
  362.883—dc23   2013045396

∞™ The paper used in this publication meets the minimum requirements of
American National Standard for Information Sciences—Permanence of Paper
for Printed Library Materials, ANSI/NISO Z39.48-1992.

Printed in the United States of America

CONTENTS

ACKNOWLEDGMENTS

As with all the titles in the Military Life series, the aim is to produce a one-stop guide that, hopefully, covers all the information you need on a specific subject. We are not trying to reinvent the wheel, simply to gather information from as many sources available as possible so that you don't have to. Almost all the information in this book comes from federal and military websites and is in the public domain. These include the Department of Defense, American Forces Press Service, U.S. Army Medical Department, Department of Veterans Affairs, Department of Health and Human Services, and the websites of all branches of the U.S. military. In particular, we would like to acknowledge the assistance given by the Military Rape Crisis Center and their permission to share case studies from their website. We have tried to extract the essentials from such public domain material. Where more information might be useful we have provided websites and resources that can help you.

INTRODUCTION

The Human Goals Charter of the Department of Defense states: "Our nation was founded on the principle that the individual has infinite dignity and worth." This is and must remain our guiding principle.

—Edwin Dorn, Under Secretary of Defense for
Personnel and Readiness, February 4, 1997

Our policy on sexual harassment is crystal clear. We believe that sexual harassment is wrong, ethically and morally. We believe it is wrong from the point of view of military discipline. And we believe it is wrong from the point of view of maintaining proper respect in the chain of command. And for all of these reasons therefore, we have a zero tolerance for sexual harassment.

—Secretary of Defense William J. Perry,
November 13, 1996

Sexual assault is a crime that takes a toll on the victim and diminishes the Department's capability by undermining core values, degrading mission readiness, potentially jeopardizing strategic alliances, and raising financial costs, according to the latest Department of Defense annual report on sexual assaults in the military, published in May 2013.

The Department seeks to reduce, with a goal to eliminate, sexual assault through institutionalized prevention efforts and policies that empower Service members to stop a sexual assault before it occurs. Sexual assault is a crime that has no place in the Department of Defense (DoD). It is an attack on the values we defend and on the cohesion our units demand, and forever changes the lives of victims and their families.

In 2005, the Department established the Sexual Assault Prevention and Response (SAPR) Program to promote prevention, encourage increased reporting of the crime, and improve response capabilities for victims. The DoD Sexual Assault Prevention and Response Office (SAPRO) is responsible for the policies that define the SAPR program and the oversight activities that assess its effectiveness. Each year it publishes an annual report, and, as the latest report reveals, little progress has been made.

Despite repeated attempts to stamp out sexual assault in the military, it has continued almost unabated. Even officials admit that the cases reported are only the tiny tip of a huge iceberg. In many cases victims are reluctant to come forward for fear of reprisals and damaging their careers. Often, the offender is the superior of the victim.

Even when victims have come forward, they have frequently been pressured to drop charges or have been quickly transferred or persuaded to leave the Service. In many cases the offender went unpunished or received nothing more than a slap on the hand. Very few were convicted of the charges made against them. Commanding officers, most of whom had little training in handling sexual assaults, frequently dismissed charges despite the evidence, for fear of damaging their unit's reputation and their own military record.

As a result, the number of sexual assaults has been steadily increasing against both serving men and women. The military's track record in handling these cases has made many victims reluctant to come forward, and even when they did, a serious lack of training throughout the chain of command has impeded how these cases were handled and frequently simply revictimized the victim.

Several highly publicized sexual assault cases over the last two years, particularly at military academies, finally caused a public outcry, and Congress decided it was time to take action. At a series of Senate and House hearings, the military's most senior officers admitted that sexual assault and harassment were ongoing major problems. With Congress threatening legislation to remove some of the military's powers to handle these cases, the Department of Defense and Chiefs of Staff promised action.

New directives have been issued spelling out how sexual assault cases are to be handled. New training methods have been introduced in all branches so that those responsible for handling such cases know their responsibilities, and new avenues of communication have been opened up to encourage more victims to come forward.

We will have to wait and see whether any of these measures have any significant effect in the months and years ahead. In all organizations employing hundreds of thousands of people, crimes will be committed, including those of a sexual nature. It is impossible to eradicate sexual assaults, but the hope must be that the new measures will seriously reduce the number of attacks and lead to a more just legal process for the victims with much more severe punishments for the perpetrators.

That is what this book is all about. It looks at the shameful history of sexual assaults in the military spanning many decades. It examines the current situation, the events that led up to the recent changes, and the attitudes of and statements from the country's most senior military leaders.

The book also details what constitutes sexual assault and harassment and then describes the many problems that victims can face as a result of being assaulted—from stress and depression to dismissal from the Service, substance abuse, and suicide. A number of case studies are given that graphically describe the impact that sexual assault has on the victim, compounded by the military's often dismissive attitude toward them.

Finally, the book looks at the new measures that have been improved for handling cases in the future, from protocols on how to investigate such cases to training at all levels. It also describes the help that is available to victims in the hope that more victims will be encouraged to come forward and receive the fair and sympathetic treatment they deserve, and that all perpetrators of such cases will be dealt with to the full extent of the law.

This book is primarily written for the victims of sexual assault and their families and friends. It explains your options as well as the physical and psychological complications that can follow an assault—and how they can be combatted. The two most important things for the victim are strong support—both from military superiors and family and friends—and seeing their attacker punished.

Another audience for this book is every serving member of the military, especially those entrusted with leadership positions. Many assaults would never have happened if a colleague had intervened when witnessing a situation getting out of hand. Everyone has a responsibility to do everything they can to prevent such an assault and not remain silent.

Finally, while this book is aimed at the military, the situations discussed are applicable in all walks of life. Sexual abuse and harassment can and do occur everywhere, especially in schools and in the workplace. The results are the same. Victims need support, but much more important is for all of us to be proactive. If we are able to step in before a perpetrator is able to commit the crime, there will be one less victim. That is a goal we should all strive for.

I

1

THE PROBLEM

The Department of Defense's 2012 Annual Report on Sexual Assault in the Military estimates that there were 26,000 sexual assaults in the military last year, up 35 percent from 19,000 in 2011, yet only 3,374 reports were filed with military police or prosecutors. Most victims are reluctant to press charges because of fear of retaliation, damage to their careers, and widespread distrust of the military justice system.

President Obama called the statistics "shameful" and "disgraceful," while Secretary of Defense Chuck Hagel labeled them a "betrayal" and a "scourge that must be stamped out."

However, analysis conducted in the documentary *The Invisible War*, directed by Kirby Dick, found that less than 1 percent of the cases resulted in a court-martial. Dick said, "500,000 uniformed men and women have been assaulted since 1991 [the year of the Navy's Tailhook sexual assaults in Las Vegas—see below], and fewer than 15 percent were ever reported."

The vast majority of cases of sexual assault and harassment are not reported because of fear of retribution from superiors and a distrust of the military investigation and court system. Another major impediment is that the officer to whom the assault has to be reported is sometimes the person who has committed the crime.

The cases that are reported are just the tip of a giant iceberg, and despite four decades of sexual harassment laws, numerous military task forces and recommendations, and a policy of zero tolerance, the situation does not appear to have improved. Some argue it has even gotten worse.

Matters came to a head early in 2013 following disclosures about sexual assault scandals at the Army's West Point Academy, the Naval Academy, and the Air Force's Joint Base San Antonio-Lackland.

In addition, an Army lieutenant colonel in charge of sexual assault prevention at Fort Campbell in Kentucky was charged with stalking and violating a restraining order obtained by his ex-wife. An Army sergeant first-class who served as a sexual assault prevention and response coordinator at Fort Hood, Texas, was charged with "abusive sexual contact, assault, pandering and maltreatment of subordinates"; and in May 2013 a lieutenant colonel in charge of the Air Force's sexual assault prevention and response branch was arrested on a charge of sexual battery.

The public outcry from the President and many others was such that sexual harassment and assault in the military because front-page news, Congress took up the issue, and military leaders pledged to take action to stamp it out.

Sexual assault in the forces constitutes a crisis in the military, the chairman of the Joint Chiefs of Staff said in a statement on May 15, 2013. "We're losing the confidence of the women who serve that we can solve this problem," Army General Martin E. Dempsey said as he returned from NATO meetings in Brussels. "That's a crisis." Dempsey has actively been researching this issue since he became the Army's Training and Doctrine Command chief in 2008. He continued the research as Army chief of staff, and now as chairman. "I tasked those around me to help me understand what a decade-plus of conflict may have done to the force," he said. "Instinctively, I knew it had to have some effect."

He said he does think the increase in sexual assaults, the rise in suicides, and the increase in instances of misconduct and indiscipline are in some way related. "This is not to make excuses," he said. "We should be better than this. In fact, we have to be better than this." All of the Joint Chiefs share his concern, Dempsey said, which was why the chiefs issued directions to the Joint Force on Sexual Assault Prevention and Response in May 2012. "That's why we are very open to some of these legislative recommendations on changing the Uniform Code of Military Justice," he said. "I just want to make sure I understand the second- and third-order of effects of them."

On June 13, 2013, Navy Secretary Ray Mabus said at a press conference that the Navy has been taking steps for years to combat the scourge of sexual assault in the ranks. He told the Defense Writers Group in Washington, DC, that two cultural barriers had to be broken down. The first culture that has to change is the "one that says this is OK, or that it is not really serious," he said. "The other is the mindset of a victim who says, 'I'm not going to report this, because nothing will happen. I won't be taken seriously, it won't be investigated, and it will hurt my career.'" The Navy is aiming resources at where it has a problem, the secretary said. The Air Force has had a problem of sexual assault at basic training, he noted, and the Navy has had a problem at its follow-on schools. The Navy has been aggressive, the Service's top civilian official said. "We're sending shore patrols out—the first time in a long time we've done that," he added. "We're stressing bystander intervention."

Congress has suggested the chain of command be removed from the prosecution of sexual assault cases. This is resisted by military leaders of branches, who argue that it "could ruin order and discipline in the ranks." In June 2013, Senator Kirsten Gillibrand (D-New York) proposed legislation that would have removed the chain of command from the prosecution of these cases and put the matter into the hands of suitably experienced legal officers. At the June Senate Armed Service Committee hearing, she told the Joint Chiefs of Staff, "Not every single commander necessarily wants women in the force, not every single commander believes what a sexual assault is, not every single commander can distinguish between a slap on the ass and a rape. You have lost the trust of the men and women who rely on you." Committee chairman Senator Carl Levin (D-Michigan) said, "The problem of sexual assault is of such scope and magnitude that it has become a stain on our military," adding that "real progress would not be seen without a cultural change in the military from the top down."

Chairman of the Joint Chiefs of Staff General Martin Dempsey, accepted that efforts to stop sexual attacks had not been successful but insisted that "reducing command responsibility could adversely affect the ability of the commander to enforce professional standards and ultimately, to accomplish the mission." Dempsey told the senators that he welcomed their input and will work closely with them. "As we consider further reforms, the role of the commander should remain central," he said. "Our goal should be to hold commanders more accountable, not render them less able to help us correct the crisis."

Army Chief of Staff General Raymond Odierno told the hearing, "We cannot legislate our way out of this problem." He acknowledged that some legal reform could be useful but added that removing the authority of commanders to handle assault cases could affect unit discipline and lead to other effects. "Without equivocation, I believe maintaining the central role of the commander in our military justice system is absolutely critical. Removing commanders, making commanders less responsible, less accountable, will not work. It will hamper the delivery of justice to the people we most want to help," he said.

Marine Corps Commandant General James F. Amos told the committee that commanding officers are the centerpiece of the Marine Corps' effectiveness as a professional and disciplined war-fighting organization. "Commanding officers are charged with establishing and training to standards and uniformly enforcing those standards," he said. "A unit will rise or fall as a direct result of the leadership of its commanding officer." They never delegate responsibility, he added, and "they should never be forced to delegate their authority."

In July 2013, Defense Secretary Chuck Hagel approved new regulations aimed at providing more support to alleged victims of sexual assault, standardizing how each Service handles cases and making sure senior commanders learn about every reported incident. Hagel's reforms require that every presiding officer at what is known as an Article 32 hearing be a lawyer. An Article 32 hearing is similar to a civilian grand jury proceeding and is held to determine whether a trial or court-martial is warranted. However, critics contend that because of its imprecise procedural rules, Article 32 hearings can be very similar to trials, with defense council allowed to subject victims to sometimes days of grueling and hostile cross-examination. Critics insist that this is yet another reason why so few victims come forward.

At the end of August 2013, the Joint Service Committee adopted a proposal—which must be endorsed by President Obama—that would afford better protections for victims testifying at Article 32 hearings. And at the time of writing, Congress was still considering a measure to take sexual abuse cases outside the victim's chain of command. Under the measure, the authority to investigate and prosecute cases would be made by impartial military prosecutors instead of senior officers with no legal training but inherent conflicts of interest.

As Senator Gillibrand said, it is time to "listen to the victims and create an independent, objective and non-biased military justice system."

SOME BACKGROUND

Within the armed forces, Executive Order 9981, signed by President Harry S. Truman on July 26, 1948, established the policy of Equality Treatment and Opportunity for all persons without regard to race, color, religion, or national origin. Additionally, it established Equal Opportunity as a fundamental principle in the armed forces of the United States.

In 1972, the Equal Employment Opportunity Commission (EEOC) was established to enforce Title VII of the 1964 Civil Rights Act. Current sexual harassment law under EEOC guidelines on discrimination because of sex, codified at 29 C.F.R. 1604.11, states the following:

> Harassment on the basis of sex is a violation of section 703 of Title VII. Unwelcome sexual advances, requests for sexual favors and other verbal or physical conduct of a sexual nature constitute sexual harassment when (1) submission to such conduct is made either explicit or implicit a term or condition of an individual's employment, (2) submission to or rejection of such conduct by an individual is used as the basis for employment decisions affecting such individual, or (3) such conduct has the purpose or effect of unreasonably interfering with an individual's work performance or creating an intimidating, hostile, or offensive working environment.

The EEOC also defined two basic requirements for sexual harassment: that the conduct in question, whether physical, verbal, or both, is unwelcome and that it is of a sexual nature. Conduct is not welcome when it is unsolicited, when the victim has done nothing to incite it, and when the victim views that conduct as undesirable or offensive. The requirement that sexually harassing conduct, whether physical or verbal, be of a sexual nature is typically fulfilled by such frequently cited behaviors as propositions, comments on the sexual areas of a woman's body, dirty jokes, pictures of nude or sexually suggestive individuals, and sexually oriented cartoons.

As a result of a number of well-publicized cases of sexual harassment in the military in the early 1990s, the Department of Defense (DoD) expanded its emphasis on the policies of sexual harassment. These incidents included the Navy's Tailhook Convention scandal and sexual assault charges at the Army's Aberdeen Proving Ground, Maryland; Fort Leonard, Missouri; and Fort Sam Houston, Texas, with drill instructors charged with sexually harassing and assaulting trainees.

In 1994, the secretary of defense (SECDEF) established a sexual harassment policy of "zero tolerance," which is the foundation used by all Military Service secretaries to provide direction and vision toward combating sexual harassment within their corps. Additionally, steps were initiated throughout all the Services to evaluate existing sexual harassment policies and modify them, if necessary, to ensure they were in compliance with the SECDEF's guidance.

Additionally, the service secretaries made significant efforts toward increasing the awareness of sexual harassment through the development of instructional guides and checklists, thus equipping commanders and super-visors with the preventive tools necessary to maintain a working environ-ment free from harassment. The service secretaries also directed an expan-sion of sexual harassment training requirements by mandating all members receive interval sexual harassment training throughout their military career.

Three task forces were established to develop three sexual harassment surveys, Forms A, B, and C. The first, Form A, replicated a 1988 survey that produced the baseline data on sexual harassment in the active-duty Ser-vices. The sole purpose of administering the Form A survey was to compare sexual harassment incident rates in 1988 and 1995. The table below outlines the results of that survey.

Table 1.1.

Type of Sexual Harassment	Women		Men	
	1988	*1995*	*1988*	*1995*
Any type	64	55	17	14
Actual/attempted rape/assault	5	4	0	0
Pressure for sexual favors	15	11	2	1
Touching, cornering	38	29	9	6
Looks, gestures	44	37	10	7
Letters, calls	14	12	3	2
Pressure for dates	26	22	3	2
Teasing, jokes	52	44	13	10
Whistles, calls	38	23	5	3
Attempts at other activities	7	7	2	2
Other attention	5	5	1	1

Unfortunately, Form A provided no opportunity for respondents to report certain types of behavior related to sexual harassment, lim-ited incidents to the workplace, and contained no items that mea-sured some areas of importance to policy makers. The 1988 survey limited the reporting of incidents to those that occurred at work. Therefore, an expanded survey, Form B, was developed to broaden the context to add experiences related to gender, including unwanted sex-related attention in situations involving (on- or off-duty; on- or off-base/post) civilian employees and contractors employed in the workplace. The main purpose of the second survey was to assess:

- what elements of the active-duty military population had unwanted experiences that they believed were gender related;

- the context, location, and circumstances under which such experiences occurred;
- the extent to which these experiences were reported and, if reported, members' satisfaction with the complaint process and response;
- the amount and effectiveness of training received by members on topics related to sexual harassment; and
- service members' views of current policies designed to prevent, reduce, or eliminate sexual harassment and of leadership commitment and progress in reducing the incidence of sexual harassment.

Administration of the Form B survey more than doubled the possible categories of reporting harassment, clearly ensuring the rates would be higher than those from the Form A and 1988 surveys.

Based on the responses to the 25 items from Form B, 43 percent of active-duty military (78 percent of women and 38 percent of men) indicated they had experienced one or more of the behaviors listed in the survey during the previous months.

Table 1.2.

Type of Sexual Harassment	Women 1995	Men 1995
Any type (one or more)	78	38
Sexual assault	6	1
Sexual coercion	13	2
Unwanted sexual attention	24	8
Sexual behavior	63	15
Crude/offensive behavior	70	35

FORM B–12995 RESULTS

A comparison of Forms A and B from 1988 to 1995 appears to show evidence that sexual harassment declined significantly in the active-duty Military Services. During this period, the percentage of women reporting incidents of sexual harassment declined nine percentage points, and the percentage of men reporting incidents declined three percentage points. Although the data appeared promising for the future of the Military Services, further analysis recognized that a considerable amount of unreported incidents and mishandling of cases and the perception of apathetic attitudes within the supervisory channels remained a major challenge for all Services.

In effect, the 1995 study and follow-ups on attitudes to leadership showed that nearly 1 in 10 women in the Army or Marine Corps had been sexually assaulted. Both surveys conducted in 1988 and 1995 also identified that 2 in 10 women reported that they were targets of "sexual coercion," which the survey defined as instances in which job benefits or losses were conditioned on sexual cooperation. The results further acknowledged that Army women had lost faith in their senior leadership's efforts and that the Marine Corps continued to have the highest rate of sexual harassment. It also found that the Navy had made the most progress since 1988, while the Air Force continued to have the lowest rate of sexual harassment. The task force concluded that only a complaints-processing system that ensured both unit effectiveness and fairness to individuals would enhance military readiness.

On May 12, 1995, the Defense Equal Opportunity Council (DEOC) task force made 48 recommendations of which 5 were to help military Equal Opportunity (EO) programs to fulfill the goals of unit effectiveness and readiness:

1. All commanders' personal commitment to EO must be visible and unequivocal.
2. DOD to establish goals, principles, and standards of performance.
3. Clear, concise, written policies to ensure that Service men and women know that discrimination and harassment are forbidden, how to recognize these offenses, how to file complaints, and how the rights of all involved will be protected.
4. EO and human relations training should continue throughout a military member's career. Training for leaders and commanders should stress their personal involvement and accountability.
5. Complaint systems should be: prompt, thorough and fair; allow informal resolution; include support services; prevent reprisals; and provide appropriate punishments.

All the recommendations were approved by the deputy secretary of defense and incorporated in DoD and Service Directives.

A review of the effects of these recommendations by USAF Major Victoria I. Bowens in 1999 (AU/ACSC/013/1999-04) found that "despite the attention and guidance provided by senior leadership in aiding operational commanders in combating sexual harassment, the issue of sexual harassment still continues to be a pervasive problem within the military environment."

A cause of concern was that the policy of "zero tolerance" was not being implemented in the way it was intended by senior leaders and "if true, is it because commanders do not understand the policy or is the concept too broad and difficult to manage?" she questioned.

That report was published 13 years ago, and little it seems has changed since then. In fact, by many accounts, the situation has deteriorated even further.

On February 4, 1997, former Secretary of the Air Force Sheila E. Widnall prepared a statement to the Senate Armed Services Committee on the Air Force's approach to ending sexual harassment. The thrust of the Air Force's policy measured up to the same level of the secretary of defense's sexual harassment policy of "zero tolerance." Simply stated, "Commanders must demonstrate visible, unequivocal leadership and personal commitment to equal opportunity, and build an organizational culture where members are valued, respected, and treated fairly."

The Air Force's policy prohibiting sexual harassment has been in existence since 1980. In 1981, the Air Force built a unit climate assessment program to help commanders assess their organization's human relations climate, which is conducted by the EO staff six months after a commander assumes command. The assessment is conducted every two years or upon request from the commander. Additionally, in May 1982, officials took a more proactive approach by giving all personnel a two-hour course in sexual harassment awareness. Two years later, the awareness program was incorporated into the human relations training, which is given to Air Force members upon the arrival of their first duty station and during professional military education. However, after the wake of the 1991 Tailhook incident, the Air Force further intensified its efforts and took an even tougher campaign against sexual harassment. Aggressive steps were taken to attack the heart of the issue:

- emphasis on commandership, selection and education for command, commander responsibilities, and personal accountability;
- continuous communication of core values to internalize for all persons the essence of the standards of the military professional;
- revision of the Air Force instruction on professional and unprofessional relationships to make clear the inherent conflict of interest in fraternization and other unprofessional relationships; and
- closer attention to the special trust and responsibilities that go with the student-teacher or trainer-trainee relationship.

These actions were not the panacea to totally eliminate sexual harassment within the Air Force; however, they moved the Air Force one step closer toward eliminating the preponderance of unprofessional behavior within its corps.

In November 1995, former Air Force Chief of Staff General Ronald R. Fogleman articulated his message to the field commanders on their commander responsibilities:

> Any conduct, in any unit, which creates a disadvantage based on race, ethnicity or gender will not be tolerated. Malicious or inappropriate behavior as well as different training standards cannot be permitted. Any indications that such behavior is occurring within a unit will prompt immediate investigation. Those responsible for such actions as well as commanders who fail to correct these problems will be held accountable.

General Fogleman further outlined four pass/fail items for Air Force leaders:

> We will not tolerate any religious, sexual or racial harassment. Period. . . . There are several reasons for this. One, it's the right thing to do. Two, it's the law of the land. The third is more fundamental. We cannot expect people to achieve their maximum potential in an environment where harassment or prejudice exists. While we're reducing resources, to include people, every person has got to be in a working environment where they can achieve their full potential.

Additionally, the Air Force established strict guidance for their wing commanders to hold Wing Climate Assessment Committee meetings at least twice a year to evaluate the overall human relations climate. Further to being the only Service with a full-time enlisted EO advisor career field, the Air Force Chief of Staff, in October 1993, directed the realignment of the Air Force Social Actions office from the Mission Support Squadron to the wing commander's staff.

The realignment now provides direct program emphasis and oversight, increases the visibility of the program, and improves the wing commander's ability to respond to EO issues affecting readiness. Not stopping there, the Air Force took a closer look at its policy statements, directives, and messages in the field addressing its EO concerns. The following major documents were published or distributed to address EO and treatment programs:

- August 11, 1994, Air Force Policy Directive 36-27, Social Actions program, provided policy guidance regarding unlawful discriminations and sexual harassment.
- August 1994, CSAF message to ALMAJCOM/CCs, sexual harassment, stated, "It is clear that our policy is zero tolerance."
- February 1995, AFPAM 36-2705, Discrimination and Sexual Harassment, for distribution to all Air Force personnel.
- November 1995, CSAF message ALMAJCOM/CCs "Command Responsibilities. Any conduct, in Any Unit, Which Creates a Disadvantage Based on Race, Ethnicity of Gender Will Not be Tolerated."
- October 1996, revised Air Force Instruction 36-2706, Military Equal Opportunity and Treatment Program. This instruction implements recommendations from the Defense Equal Opportunity Council Task Force on Discrimination and Sexual Harassment.
- 1999, revised AFI 36-2909, Professional and Unprofessional Relationships.

Further addressed within AFI 36-2706 is guidance to include the complaint-processing procedures and grievance channels and processes, and procedures and responsibilities of commanders and personnel to resolve complaints at the lowest level. The AFI delineates responsibilities as follows:

- The responsibilities of the wing commander are to provide an environment free from discrimination and harassment, review all closed discrimination cases monthly.
- Unlawful discrimination or sexual harassment cases involving senior officials, general officers, and Senior Executive Service (SES) equivalents are immediately forwarded and reported to the AF Inspector General in the Office of the Secretary of the Air Force. Cases involving colonels or colonel selects must also be reported to the IG.
- Reprisal complaints are immediately referred to the IG. Reprisal protection is mandated by law, DoD directive and AF Instruction.

An Air Force Inspector General fraud, waste, and abuse hotline has always been available, whose sole purpose is to accept and investigate concerns expressed by Air Force members.

However, a specific sexual harassment "1-800" hotline established by the Headquarters Air Force Personnel Center reinforced the Air Force's commitment to investigate equal opportunity and treatment complaints. Qualified Equal Opportunity Treatment (EOT) personnel staff the hotline.

According to a nine-month-long investigation conducted by the *Denver Post* and published as a special report in 2004:

> As many as 20,000 women have been sexually assaulted while serving in the armed forces Over the past decade, nearly 5,000 accused Army sex offenders avoided prosecution More than 10,000 cases of spouse abuse were substantiated annually between 1997 and 2001. In 2,000 12,068 cases of spouse abuse were reported; only 26 led to courts-martial Victims lack support services, and many are left vulnerable to pressure and intimidation from commanders and peers.

The full report, which contains scores of sexual assault and domestic abuse cases, can be found at http://extras.denverpost.com/justice/tdp_betrayal.pdf.

IF YOU ARE THE VICTIM OF A SEXUAL ASSAULT

Go to a safe location away from the attacker.

Call 877-995-5247 or text a location or zip code to 55-247 (within CONUS) or 202-470-5546 (OCONUS) or online chat with a counselor at www.SafeHelpline.org 24 hours a day or contact your local sexual assault response coordinator (SARC), victim advocate (VA), or healthcare provider.

You may also contact your chain of command or law enforcement (military or civilian); however, if you do, an investigation will occur and you will not have the option of making a Restricted Report (see below).

Seek medical care as soon as possible. Even if you do not have any visible physical injuries, you may be at risk of becoming pregnant or acquiring a sexually transmitted disease. Ask the healthcare provider to conduct a sexual assault forensic examination (SAFE) to preserve forensic evidence. If you suspect you have been drugged, request that a urine sample be collected.

Preserve all evidence of the assault. Do not bathe, wash your hands, eat or drink, or brush your teeth. Do not clean or straighten up the crime scene.

Write down, tape, or record by any other means all the details you can recall about the assault and your assailant.

2

CATEGORIES OF
SEXUAL HARASSMENT

a. *Verbal.* Examples of verbal sexual harassment may include telling sexual jokes; using sexually explicit profanity, threats, sexually oriented cadences, or sexual comments; whistling in a sexually suggestive manner; and describing certain attributes of one's physical appearance in a sexual manner. Verbal sexual harassment may also include using terms of endearment such as "honey," "babe," "sweetheart," "dear," "stud," or "hunk" in referring to soldiers, civilian coworkers, or family members.
b. *Nonverbal.* Examples of nonverbal sexual harassment may include staring at someone (that is, "undressing someone with one's eyes"), blowing kisses, winking, or licking one's lips in a suggestive manner. Nonverbal sexual harassment also includes printed material (e.g., displaying sexually oriented pictures or cartoons); using sexually oriented screen savers on one's computer; or sending sexually oriented notes, letters, faxes, or e-mail.
c. *Physical contact.* Examples of physical sexual harassment may include touching, patting, pinching, bumping, grabbing, cornering, or blocking a passageway; kissing; and providing unsolicited back or neck rubs. Sexual assault and rape are extreme forms of sexual harassment and serious criminal acts.

TYPES OF SEXUAL HARASSMENT

a. *Quid pro quo.* "Quid pro quo" is a Latin term meaning "this for that." This term refers to conditions placed on a person's career or terms of employment in return for favors. It includes implicit or explicit threats of adverse action if the person does not submit to such conditions and

15

promises of favorable actions if the person does submit to such conditions. Examples include demanding sexual favors in exchange for a promotion, award, or favorable assignment; disciplining or relieving a subordinate who refuses sexual advances; and threats of poor job evaluation for refusing sexual advances. Incidents of "quid pro quo" may also have a harassing effect on third persons. It may result in allegations of sexual favoritism or general discrimination when a person feels unfairly deprived of recognition, advancement, or career opportunities because of favoritism shown to another soldier or civilian employee on the basis of a sexual relationship. An example would be a soldier who is not recommended for promotion and who believes that his or her squad leader recommended another soldier in his or her squad for promotion on the basis of provided or promised sexual favors, not upon merit or ability.

b. *Hostile environment.* A hostile environment occurs when soldiers or civilians are subjected to offensive, unwanted, and unsolicited comments or behaviors of a sexual nature. If these behaviors unreasonably interfere with their performance, regardless of whether the harasser and the victim are in the same workplace, then the environment is classified as hostile. A hostile environment brings the topic of sex or gender differences into the workplace in any one of a number of forms. It does not necessarily include the more blatant acts of "quid pro quo"; it normally includes nonviolent, gender-biased sexual behaviors (e.g., the use of derogatory gender-biased terms, comments about body parts, suggestive pictures, explicit jokes, and unwanted touching).

Pursuant to the legislated requirements, the following terms are used by the Services for annual and quarterly reporting of the dispositions of subjects in sexual assault investigations conducted by the MCIO. Services must adapt their investigative policies and procedures to comply with these terms.

Substantiated Reports. Dispositions in this category come from Unrestricted Reports that have been investigated and found to have sufficient evidence to provide to command for consideration of action to take some form of punitive, corrective, or discharge action against an offender.

(1) Substantiated Reports against Service Member Subjects. A substantiated report of sexual assault is an Unrestricted Report that was investigated by an MCIO, provided to the appropriate military command for consideration of action, and found to have sufficient evidence to support the command's action against the subject. Actions against

the subject may include initiation of a court-martial, nonjudicial punishment, administrative discharge, and other adverse administrative actions that result from a report of sexual assault or associated misconduct (e.g., adultery, housebreaking, false official statement).

(2) Substantiated Reports by Service Member Victims. A substantiated report of a sexual assault victim's Unrestricted Report that was investigated by an MCIO, provided to the appropriate military command for consideration of action, and found to have sufficient evidence to support the command's action against the subject. However, there are instances where an Unrestricted Report of sexual assault by a Service member victim may be substantiated but the command is not able to take action against the person who is the subject of the investigation. These categories include the following: the subject of the investigation could not be identified; the subject died or deserted from the Service before action could be taken; the subject was a civilian or foreign national not subject to the UCMJ; or the subject was a Service member being prosecuted by a civilian or foreign authority.

Substantiated Report Disposition Descriptions. In the event of several types of action a commander takes against the same offender, only the most serious action taken is reported, as provided for in the following list, in descending order of seriousness. For each offender, any court-martial sentence and nonjudicial punishment administered by commanders pursuant to Article 15 of the UCMJ is reported annually to the DoD in the case synopses or via DSAID. Further additional actions of a less serious nature in the descending list should also be included in the case synopses reported to the Department. Reference (k) of Article 15 requires the reporting of the number of victims associated with each of the following disposition categories.

1. Commander Action for Sexual Assault Offense
   (a) Type (a) Court-Martial Charges Preferred (Initiated) for Sexual Assault Offense. A court-martial charge was preferred (initiated) for at least one of the offenses punishable by Articles 120 and 125 of the UCMJ, or an attempt to commit an Article 120 or 125 UCMJ offense that would be charged as a violation of Article 80 of the UCMJ. (See Rules for Courts-Martial 307 and 401 of Reference [q].)
   (b) Nonjudicial Punishments (Article 15, UCMJ). Disciplinary action for at least one of the UCMJ offenses comprised within the

SAPR definition of sexual assault that was initiated pursuant to Article 15 of the UCMJ.

(c) Administrative Discharges. Commander action taken to involuntarily separate the offender from military service that is based in whole or in part on an offense within the SAPR definition of sexual assault.

(d) Other Adverse Administrative Actions. In the absence of an administrative discharge action, any other administrative action that was initiated (including corrective measures such as counseling, admonition, reprimand, exhortation, disapproval, criticism, censure, reproach, rebuke, extra military instruction, or other administrative withholding of privileges, or any combination thereof), and that is based in whole or in part on an offense within the SAPR definition of sexual assault. Cases should be placed in this category only when an administrative action other than an administrative discharge is the only action taken. If an "other administrative action" is taken in combination with another more serious action (e.g., court-martial, nonjudicial punishment, administrative discharge, or civilian or foreign court action), only report the case according to the more serious action taken.

Commander Action for Other Criminal Offense. Report actions against subjects in this category when there is probable cause for an offense, but only for a nonsexual assault offense (i.e., the commander took action on a nonsexual assault offense because an investigation showed that the allegations did not meet the required elements of, or there was insufficient evidence for, any of the UCMJ offenses that constitute the SAPR definition of sexual assault). Instead, an investigation disclosed other offenses arising from the sexual assault allegation or incident that met the required elements of, and there was sufficient evidence for, another offense under the UCMJ. Report court-martial charges preferred, nonjudicial punishments, and sentences imposed in the case synopses provided to the DoD. To comply with Reference (k), the number of victims associated with each of the following categories must also be reported.

(a) Court-martial charges preferred (initiated) for a nonsexual assault offense.

(b) Nonjudicial punishments (Article 15, UCMJ) for nonsexual assault offense.

(c) Administrative discharges for nonsexual assault offense.

(d) Other adverse administrative actions for nonsexual assault offense.

Command Action Precluded. Dispositions reported in this category come from an Unrestricted Report that was investigated by an MCIO and provided to the appropriate military command for consideration of action, but the evidence did not support taking action against the subject of the investigation because the victim declined to participate in the military justice action, there was insufficient evidence of any offense to take command action, the report was unfounded by command, the victim died prior to completion of the military justice action, or the statute of limitations for the alleged offense(s) expired. Reference (k) requires the reporting of the number of victims associated with each of the following disposition categories.

(1) Victim Declined to Participate in the Military Justice Action. Commander action is precluded or declined because the victim has declined to further cooperate with military authorities or prosecutors in a military justice action.

(2) Insufficient Evidence for Prosecution. Although the allegations made against the alleged offender meet the required elements of at least one criminal offense listed in the SAPR definition of sexual assault (see Reference [b]), there was insufficient evidence to legally prove those elements beyond a reasonable doubt and proceed with the case. (If the reason for concluding that there is insufficient evidence is that the victim declined to cooperate, then the reason for being unable to take action should be entered as "victim declined to participate in the military justice action," and not entered as "insufficient evidence.")

(3) Victim's Death. Victim died before completion of the military justice action.

(4) Statute of Limitations Expired. Determination that, pursuant to Article 43 of the UCMJ, the applicable statute of limitations has expired and the case may not be prosecuted.

Command Action Declined. Dispositions in this category come from an Unrestricted Report that was investigated by an MCIO and provided to the appropriate military command for consideration of action, but the commander determined the report was unfounded as to the allegations against the subject of the investigation. Unfounded allegations reflect a determination by command, with the supporting advice of a qualified legal officer, that the allegations made against the alleged offender did not occur nor were attempted. These cases are either false or baseless. Reference (k) requires the reporting of the number of victims associated with this category.

(1) False Cases. Evidence obtained through an investigation shows that an offense was not committed nor attempted by the subject of the investigation.

(2) Baseless Cases. Evidence obtained through an investigation shows that an alleged offense did not meet at least one of the required elements of a UCMJ offense constituting the SAPR definition of sexual assault or was improperly reported as a sexual assault.

Subject outside DoD's Legal Authority. When the subject of the investigation or the action being taken is beyond DoD's jurisdictional authority or ability to act, use the following descriptions to report case disposition. To comply with Reference (k), Services must also identify the number of victims associated with these dispositions and specify when there was insufficient evidence that an offense occurred in the following categories.

(1) Offender Is Unknown. The investigation is closed because no person could be identified as the alleged offender.

(2) Subject is a Civilian or Foreign National Not Subject to UCMJ. The subject of the investigation is not amenable to military UCMJ jurisdiction for action or disposition.

(3) Civilian or Foreign Authority is Prosecuting Service Member. A civilian or foreign authority has the sexual assault allegation for action or disposition, even though the alleged offender is also subject to the UCMJ.

(4) Offender Died or Deserted. Commander action is precluded because of the death or desertion of the alleged offender or subject of the investigation.

Report Unfounded by MCIO. Determination by the MCIO that the allegations made against the alleged offender did not occur nor were attempted. These cases are either false or baseless. Reference (k) requires the reporting of the number of victims associated with this category.

(1) False Cases. Evidence obtained through an MCIO investigation shows that an offense was not committed nor attempted by the subject of the investigation.

(2) Baseless Cases. Evidence obtained through an investigation shows that alleged offense did not meet at least one of the required elements of a UCMJ offense constituting the SAPR definition of sexual assault or was improperly reported as a sexual assault.

HAZING

Hazing is another subject that every branch of the military takes very seriously and is working diligently to stamp out. Hazing is often regarded as a required rite of passage, but it can lead to serious assault, both physical and sexual, and in some cases even death. There have been a number of high-profile hazing cases in recent months. Last year two members of the military committed suicide after allegedly being hazed in separate attacks. One was a Marine and the other a soldier, both serving in Afghanistan.

While all branches of the military condemn hazing and have policies against it, the practice continues. Now Congress has started a series of hearings to examine the scope of the problem and what the Pentagon is doing to stop it.

Marine Corps Commandant General Jim Amos has called for a full review of the Corp's 15-year-old policy on hazing, has ordered that all hazing allegations be tracked and investigated, and has told senior officers to be more aggressive in tackling claims of abuse.

"Regardless of the form it takes, hazing is always unacceptable. It destroys our Marines' confidence and trust in their fellow Marines and in unit leadership, thus undermining unit cohesion and combat readiness," Amos wrote in a letter to the Corps. Unfortunately, there are few details about how widespread the problem is. When Department of Defense officials were asked by members of Congress for hazing statistics, they were unable to produce any figures. The Pentagon is trying to get this information from each branch of the military, although it is not clear whether every Service documents hazing allegations.

In evidence to the House committee on March 22, 2012, U.S. Coast Guard Master Chief Petty Officer Michael Leavitt said,

> As the Master Chief Petty Officer of the Coast Guard ensuring our personnel are treated with dignity and respect is a responsibility I take very seriously.
>
> The Coast Guard does not tolerate hazing. Hazing is contrary to our core values of honor, respect and devotion to duty and the nature of our missions.
>
> The Coast Guard has published a clear and unambiguous policy prohibiting hazing, including requirements for initial training of all Military Service members, as well as annual training thereafter. When hazing has occurred our policy requires that offenders are held accountable. All Commanding Officers are required to investigate any hazing incident and initiate appropriate action to hold those accountable for hazing

misconduct, as well as to ensure accountability within the chain of command if hazing was condoned.

The Coast Guard defines hazing as any physical, verbal, or psychological conduct in which a military member causes another military member to suffer or to be exposed to any cruel, abusive, humiliating, oppressive, demeaning, or harmful activity, regardless of the perpetrator's and recipient's Service or rank. Soliciting or coercing another to conduct such activity also constitutes hazing.

The Coast Guard's hazing policy is found in the Discipline and Conduct Manual. The policy defines hazing, outlines roles and responsibilities, mandates annual training, and lists consequences. Furthermore, the policy clearly states that consent by the hazing victim does not obviate accountability of either the persons doing the hazing or the Command that condones or facilitates a hazing incident. Hazing incidents can be adjudicated under the provisions of the Uniform Code of Military Justice. Depending on the severity of the hazing incident, and how it is disposed of, punishment may include confinement, fines, reduction in rank, and/or punitive discharge from the Coast Guard.

Similar to hazing, prohibited harassment policy is found in the Coast Guard's Civil Rights Manual. Prohibited harassment is defined as including, but not limited to, unwelcome conduct, whether verbal, nonverbal, or physical conduct, that has the purpose or effect of unreasonably interfering with an individual's work performance or creating an intimidating, offensive, or hostile environment on the basis of an individual's protected status, which includes: race, color, religion, sex, national origin, age, disability, genetic information, sexual orientation, marital status, parental status, political affiliation, or any other basis protected by law. While hazing and prohibited harassment are similar, each type of case is reported and acted upon in a different manner. In each case, perpetrators are subject to prompt disciplinary action, including discharge and other actions authorized under the Uniform Code of Military Justice. Incidents of prohibited harassment are processed in accordance with the Coast Guard's Anti-harassment and Hate Incident Procedures and as a complaint of employment discrimination pursuant to the Coast Guard's Civil Rights Manual.

"Hazing typically occurs in connection with unofficial, unsupervised initiations or other informal 'rites of passage' that are not authorized in the Coast Guard. Traditional ceremonies are permitted but must be conducted with proper command sanction and oversight to prevent harassment of any kind," said Leavitt.

"Assault and Sexual Assault are specific illegal acts defined in the Uniform Code of Military Justice and could potentially be committed during incidences of hazing. Incidences of assault or sexual assault occurring as part of hazing are aggravating factors, and therefore carry the potential for more severe consequences to offenders."

In February 2010, the Coast Guard Investigative Service concluded a nearly yearlong investigation into allegations that former crew members onboard Coast Guard Cutter *Venturous*, home ported in St. Petersburg, Florida, had engaged in hazing between the summer of 2007 and the spring of 2009. As a result of the investigation, seven Coast Guardsmen were tried by courts-martial for the most serious misconduct related to hazing activities. Several other crew members received administrative action under the Uniform Code of Military Justice for less serious infractions. According to court records, the hazing took place in the berthing areas of the ship while underway and was done unbeknownst to senior leadership. The seven courts-martial resulted in five members receiving confinement or restrictions of up to five months, six members being reduced in pay grade, three members forfeiting pay, one member being discharged, and one member receiving a Bad Conduct Discharge.

In addition to the hazing on *Venturous*, there have been three additional courts-martial stemming from hazing incidents since 2009. These included cases at Station Cape Disappointment, SECTOR Mobile, and SECTOR San Francisco. Twenty-three Coast Guardsmen have been identified as the "targets," or victims of serious hazing misconduct. Eighteen, or 78 percent, of the victims are Caucasian. Other victims are distributed across many racial profiles, including one Asian American, one African American, one Hispanic, one Hawaiian Islander, and one Native American/Alaska Native. "Juniority" of rank appears to be the common characteristic of the victims of serious hazing misconduct.

Hazing Victim Racial Profiles

White	Asian	Black	Hispanic	Other	Total
78% (18)	4% (1)	4% (1)	4% (1)	4% (1)	23

No data is available to determine if hazing was or was not a contributing factor in any suicide that has occurred in the Coast Guard. Throughout the past ten years, the number of suicides has remained fairly consistent, averaging six active-duty and reservist suicides per year, which represents roughly 0.01 percent of our workforce.

Sergeant Major of the Army Raymond Chandler, speaking at the House Armed Forces Committee's military personal subcommittee, Washington, DC, March 22, 2012, said, "My overall message to the force is the Army profession. I talk about what it means to be a professional, how Soldiers should conduct themselves, and more importantly, how they should treat each other." Master Chief Petty Officer of the Navy Rick West told the committee that "people are absolutely our most precious asset. Their individual success and the Navy's collective mission accomplishment lie in our ability to provide an environment that promotes inclusiveness and a validated sense of value to the team." "Hazing unequivocally destroys these ideas and is not tolerated in your Navy," West said. "It is inconsistent to our core values of honor, courage and commitment, and detrimental to individual esteem and unit cohesion."

Sergeant Major of the Marine Corps Michael P. Barrett stated, "Hazing is not a part of our service culture or who we are."

> Hazing fosters a climate of maltreatment and cruelty—concepts inconsistent with our core values. As an institution, the only way that the Marine Corps can exist, survive and thrive is through fostering a climate where Marines have every opportunity for participation and advancement in accordance with their talents, backgrounds, culture and skills.

HOW TO TACKLE THE PROBLEM

Preventing hazing can best be achieved by addressing two key elements: training and leadership. Awareness and support of the hazing policies are emphasized by senior leadership through the use of communications to all ranks and other formal and informal outreach efforts. For example, the Coast Guard commandant as well as the Pacific and Atlantic Area commanders released official messages regarding the responsibility of all Coast Guardsmen to comply with the Coast Guard's zero tolerance hazing policy. The commandant included a requirement in his message that all commanding officers and officers in charge read the message at the next quarters or appropriate muster to ensure that his expectations and intent are clear. Training courses held at the Leadership Development Center for Prospective Commanding Officers and Boat Forces Command Cadre include segments on hazing, aiming to ensure future leaders understand and enforce the policy.

Hazing prevention cannot be achieved purely by the actions of military leaders. All personnel must understand that hazing will not be tolerated and no one may consent to being hazed. To ensure awareness throughout the military workforce, most branches provide initial training on hazing to all new recruits and require annual unit training.

3

IMPEDIMENTS TO REPORTING

Sexual assault is the most underreported crime in our society and in the military. While the Department of Defense prefers complete reporting of sexual assaults to activate both victims' services and law enforcement actions, it recognizes that some victims desire only medical and support services and no command or law enforcement involvement. The Department believes its first priority is for victims to be protected; to be treated with dignity and respect; and to receive the medical treatment, care, and counseling that they deserve. Under DoD's confidentiality policy, sexual assault victims are offered two reporting options—Restricted Reporting and Unrestricted Reporting.

DoD's confidentiality policy permits victims of sexual assault to report the crime to specified individuals who can then ensure the victim receives medical care, treatment, and counseling without notifying command or law enforcement officials. Covered individuals include the sexual assault response coordinator (SARC); victim advocates (VA); healthcare providers; and chaplains. For purposes of public safety and command responsibility, the SARC will notify the installation commander that an assault has occurred and provide details that will not identify the victim. (See Directive-Type Memorandum, Confidentiality Policy for Victims of Sexual Assault [JTF-SAPR-009], for complete details.)

This policy provides victims some personal space and time, and increased control over the release and management of their personal information. This hopefully empowers them to seek relevant information and support to make more informed decisions about participating in the criminal investigation. Jurisdictions with similar policies have found that confidentiality actually leads to increased reporting rates. Even if the victim chooses not to pursue an official investigation, this additional reporting avenue gives commanders a clearer picture of the sexual violence within their command, and enhances a commander's ability to provide an environment that is safe and contributes to the well-being and mission-readiness of all of its members.

RESTRICTED REPORTING

This option is recommended for victims of sexual assault who wish to confidentially disclose the crime to specifically identified individuals and receive medical treatment and counseling without triggering the official investigative process. Service members who are sexually assaulted and desire Restricted Reporting under this policy must report the assault to a SARC, VA, or healthcare provider.

As provided for above, victims may also discuss the assault with a chaplain. Discussing the assault with a chaplain is not a Restricted Report under this policy; it is a communication that may be protected under the military rules of evidence (MRE) or applicable statues and regulations. The Restricted Reporting process does not affect any privilege recognized under the MRE. This policy on Restricted Reporting is in addition to the current protections afforded by privileged communications with a chaplain, and does not alter or affect those protections.

Healthcare providers will initiate the appropriate care and treatment, and report the sexual assault to the SARC in lieu of reporting it to law enforcement or the command. Upon notification of a reported sexual assault, the SARC will immediately assign a VA to the victim. The assigned VA will provide accurate information on the process of Restricted versus Unrestricted Reporting.

At the victim's discretion/request an appropriately trained healthcare provider shall conduct a sexual assault forensic examination (SAFE), which may include the collection of evidence. In the absence of a DoD provider, the service member will be referred to an appropriate civilian facility for the SAFE.

Who May Make a Restricted Report

Restricted Reporting is available at this time only to military personnel of the Armed Forces and the Coast Guard. Military personnel include members on active duty and members of the Reserve component (Reserve and National Guard) provided they are performing federal duty (active-duty training or inactive-duty training and members of the National Guard in federal [Title 10] status). Members of the Reserve component not performing federal duty are not eligible. Retired members of any component are not eligible. Dependents are not eligible. DoD civilian employees are not eligible. Restricted reports may be made any time on or after June 14, 2005.

Example of Restricted Reporting

Service member Smith arrives at the base medical emergency room and reports she has been sexually assaulted. Healthcare providers immediately notify the SARC and begin any appropriate emergency medical treatment.

The SARC assigns a VA to assist service member Smith. The VA meets service member Smith at the hospital and explains the Unrestricted/Restricted Reporting options and the processes associated with each, to include applicable pros/cons.

Service member Smith elects the Restricted Reporting option.

Service member Smith is asked if she would like a forensic examination, and she agrees.

The VA advises the healthcare provider that service member Smith has elected the Restricted Reporting option and would like a SAFE.

Forensic evidence of the assault is collected and preserved in a non-personally identifying manner.

The healthcare provider determines and schedules follow-up medical treatment as appropriate.

The VA advises the SARC that service member Smith has elected the Restricted Reporting option.

Within 24 hours of service member Smith's Restricted Report, the SARC will inform the installation commander that an assault has occurred, and provide the commander with nonidentifying personal information/details related to the sexual assault allegation. This information includes: rank; gender; age; race; service; date; time; and/or location. Information is disclosed in a manner that preserves the victim's anonymity. Careful consideration of which details to include is of particular significance at installations or other locations where there are a limited number of minority females or female officers assigned.

The installation commander may notify the criminal investigators. However, no criminal investigation will be initiated unless originated from another source or the victim elects to come forward via Unrestricted Reporting. The installation commander identifies trends and takes appropriate measures (i.e., increased security patrols, enhanced education and training, enhanced environmental and safety measures) to prevent further sexual assaults.

The SARC maintains information regarding the number of sexual assaults for both Unrestricted and Restricted Reports. Restricted Report numbers will be included in the annual report. The SARC will also capture trends and perform trend analysis. SARC awareness of trends will be a first line of defense against a potential serial assailant. The SARC can at any time return to service member Smith to ask if she is willing to reconsider her Restricted Reporting decision given the potential of a serial offender.

The VA maintains communication and contact with the victim as needed for continued victim support.

Considerations When Electing a Restricted Reporting Decision

BENEFITS

You receive appropriate medical treatment, advocacy, and counseling.

Provides some personal space and time to consider your options and to begin the healing process.

Empowers you to seek relevant information and support to make more informed decisions about participating in the criminal investigation.

You control the release and management of your personal information.

You decide whether and when to move forward with initiating an investigation.

LIMITATIONS

Your assailant remains unpunished and capable of assaulting other victims.

You cannot receive a military protective order.

You will continue to have contact with your assailant, if he/she is in your organization or billeted with you.

Evidence from the crime scene where the assault occurred will be lost, and the official investigation, should you switch to an Unrestricted Report, will likely encounter significant obstacles.

You will not be able to discuss the assault with anyone, to include your friends, without imposing an obligation on them to report the crime. The only exceptions would be chaplains, designated health-care providers, your assigned victim advocate, and the sexual assault response coordinator.

You will be ineligible to invoke the collateral misconduct provision of the Department's sexual assault policy in the event that your command learns that you had been engaged in some form of misconduct at the time you were assaulted.

UNRESTRICTED REPORTING

This option is recommended for victims of sexual assault who desire medical treatment, counseling, and an official investigation of the crime. When selecting Unrestricted Reporting, you should use current reporting channels, e.g. chain of command or law enforcement; report the incident to the SARC; or request healthcare providers to notify law enforcement. Upon notification of a reported sexual assault, the SARC will immediately assign a VA. At the victim's discretion/request, the healthcare provider shall conduct a SAFE, which may include the collection of evidence. Details regarding the incident will be limited to only those personnel who have a legitimate need to know.

Unrestricted Reporting Example

Service member Smith arrives at the base medical emergency room and reports she has been sexually assaulted. Healthcare providers immediately notify the SARC and begin administration of any emergency medical treatment as appropriate.

The SARC assigns a VA to assist service member Smith. The VA meets service member Smith at the hospital, explains the Unrestricted/Restricted Reporting options, and processes associated with each to include applicable pros/cons.

Service member Smith elects the Unrestricted Reporting option.

The VA immediately notifies the appropriate criminal investigative service and the victim's unit commander.

Criminal investigators arrive and begin the investigation.

Service member Smith is asked if she would like a SAFE, and she agrees.

The VA advises the healthcare provider that service member Smith has elected the Unrestricted Reporting option and would like a SAFE.

Forensic evidence of the assault is collected by healthcare providers, and at its conclusion, criminal investigators take chain of custody.

The healthcare provider determines and schedules follow-up medical treatment as appropriate.

The VA advises the SARC that service member Smith has elected the Unrestricted Reporting option.

In addition to any current existing channels of notification, within 24 hours of service member Smith's Unrestricted Report, the SARC will inform the installation commander that an assault has occurred and provide the commander with the details of the assault.

The SARC maintains information regarding the number of sexual assaults for both Unrestricted and Restricted Reports. Restricted Report numbers will be included in the annual report. The SARC will also capture trends and perform trend analysis.

The VA maintains communications and contact with victim as needed for continued support.

The DoD seeks increased reporting by victims of sexual assault. A system that is perceived as fair and treats victims with dignity and respect, and promotes privacy and confidentiality, may have a positive impact in bringing victims forward to provide information about being assaulted. The Restricted Reporting option is intended to give victims additional time and increased control over the release and management of their personal information and empowers them to seek relevant information and support to make more informed decisions about participating in the criminal investigation. A victim who receives support, appropriate care, and treatment, and is provided an opportunity to make an informed decision about a criminal investigation is more likely to develop increased trust that the victim's needs are of concern to the command. As a result, this trust may eventually lead the victim to decide to pursue an investigation and convert the Restricted Report to an Unrestricted Report.

Impact of Underreporting

Underreporting of sexual assault interferes with the Department's ability to provide victims with needed care and hinders the Department in holding offenders appropriately accountable. Much remains to be done to improve reporting, as DoD estimates indicate the majority of victims experiencing unwanted sexual contact (USC) do not make a sexual assault report.

However, with the SAPR program implementation in 2005, there has been a 98 percent increase in the number of sexual assaults reported to the Department. Each year, the Department receives reports of sexual assault from both military and civilian victims. The Department responds to all reports of sexual assault, but it looks to the number of service member victims in sexual assault reports as a key metric of program progress. Since the SAPR program was implemented, the number of service members accounted for in reports of sexual assault has increased by 131 percent.

Although reports to DoD authorities are unlikely to account for all USCs estimated to occur in a given year, it is the Department's intent to narrow this gap and reduce the underreporting of sexual assault in the military community.

4

SEXUAL ASSAULT
AND MENTAL HEALTH

MST AND ITS EFFECTS

"Military sexual trauma" (MST) is the term that the Department of Veterans Affairs uses to refer to sexual assault or repeated, threatening sexual harassment that occurred while the veteran was in the military. It includes any sexual activity where someone is involved against his or her will—he or she may have been pressured into sexual activities (e.g., with threats of negative consequences for refusing to be sexually cooperative or with implied faster promotions or better treatment in exchange for sex), may have been unable to consent to sexual activities (e.g., when intoxicated), or may have been physically forced into sexual activities. Other experiences that fall into the category of MST include unwanted sexual touching or grabbing; threatening, offensive remarks about a person's body or sexual activities; and/or threatening or unwelcome sexual advances.

Both women and men can experience MST during their service. All veterans seen at Veterans Health Administration (VHA) facilities are asked about experiences of sexual trauma, because we know that any type of trauma can affect a person's physical and mental health, even many years later. We also know that people can recover from trauma. The VA has free services to help veterans do this. You do not need to have a VA disability rating (be "service connected") to receive these services and may be able to receive services even if you are not eligible for other VA care. You do not need to have reported the incident(s) when they happened or have other documentation that they occurred.

Information about how commonly MST occurs comes from VA's universal screening program. Under this program, all veterans seen at VHA facilities are asked whether they experienced sexual trauma during their military service; veterans who respond "yes" are asked if they are interested in learning about MST-related services available. Not every veteran who responds "yes" needs or is necessarily interested in treatment. It's important to note that rates obtained from VA screening cannot be used to make any estimate of the rate of MST among all those serving in the U.S. Military, as they are drawn only from veterans who have chosen to seek VA health care. Also, a positive response does not indicate that the perpetrator was a member of the military.

About 1 in 5 women and 1 in 100 men seen in VHA facilities respond "yes" when screened for MST. Though rates of MST are higher among women, because of the disproportionate ratio of men to women in the military there are actually only slightly fewer men seen in VHA facilities that have experienced MST than there are women.

Safe Helpline

The DoD has launched the Safe Helpline, a groundbreaking crisis support service for members of the DoD community affected by sexual assault. Safe Helpline provides live, one-on-one support and information to the worldwide DoD community.

The service is confidential, anonymous, secure, and available worldwide, 24/7, by click, call, or text—providing victims with the help they need, anytime, anywhere. Specially trained Safe Helpline staff provide help three ways.

ONLINE HELPLINE

Safe Helpline provides live, confidential help through a secure instant-messaging format at SafeHelpline.org. The website also contains vital information about recovering from and reporting a sexual assault.

TELEPHONE HELPLINE

Safe Helpline also provides live, confidential help over the phone—just call. The telephone helpline is available from anywhere, anytime—24/7, worldwide: 877-995-5247. The phone number is the same inside the United States or via the Defense Switched Network (DSN). When calling from the DSN, there are four toll-free area codes (800, 888, 866, and 877) to enable a direct dialing capability. DSN users can dial U.S. toll-free numbers by simply dialing 94 + the 10-digit toll-free number.

The Telephone Helpline staff even transfer callers to installation and base SARCs, Military OneSource, the National Suicide Prevention Lifeline, and civilian sexual assault service providers.

Safe Helpline can provide you with referrals by text to your mobile phone. You can text your zip code, installation, or base name to 55-247 (inside the United States) or 202-470-5546 (outside the United States), and Safe Helpline will text back contact information for the SARC on your installation or base. You can also search for help here.

Safe Helpline services (click, call, or text) are administered by the DoD SAPRO and are operated by RAINN (Rape, Abuse & Incest National Network), the nation's largest anti-sexual violence organization. However, your information will remain confidential. RAINN will not share your name or any other personally identifying information with SAPRO or your chain of command.

RAINN created and operates the National Sexual Assault Hotline (800-656-HOPE) in partnership with over 1,100 local rape crisis centers nationwide. RAINN also runs the National Sexual Assault Online Hotline (online.rainn.org). Together, the hotlines have helped more than 1.6 million people since 1994.

How Can MST Affect Veterans?

When overwhelmed by strong emotions, the body and mind sometimes react by shutting down and becoming numb. As a result, veterans may have difficulty experiencing loving feelings or feeling some emotions, especially when upset by traumatic memories. Like many of the other reactions to trauma, this emotional numbing reaction is not something the veteran is doing on purpose.

It's important to remember that MST is an experience, not a diagnosis or a mental health condition in and of itself. Given the range of distressing sexually related experiences that veterans report, it is not surprising that there are a wide range of emotional reactions that veterans have in response to these events. Even after severely distressing experiences, there is no one way that everyone will respond—the type, severity, and duration of a veteran's difficulties will all vary based on factors like whether he/she has a prior history of abuse, the types of responses from others he/she received at the time of the experiences, and whether the experience happened once or was repeated over time. For some veterans, experiences of MST may continue to affect their mental and physical health, even many years later.

Some of the difficulties both female and male survivors of MST may have include:

Strong emotions: feeling depressed; having intense, sudden emotional reactions to things; feeling angry or irritable all the time

Feelings of numbness: feeling emotionally "flat," difficulty experiencing emotions like love or happiness

Trouble sleeping: trouble falling or staying asleep; disturbing nightmares

Difficulties with attention, concentration, and memory: trouble staying focused; frequently finding their mind wandering; having a hard time remembering things

Problems with alcohol or other drugs: drinking to excess or using drugs daily; getting intoxicated or "high" to cope with memories or emotional reactions; drinking to fall asleep

Difficulty with things that remind them of their experiences of sexual trauma: feeling on edge or "jumpy" all the time; difficulty feeling safe; going out of their way to avoid reminders of their experiences; difficulty trusting others

Difficulties in relationships: feeling isolated or disconnected from others; abusive relationships; trouble with employers or authority figures

Physical health problems: sexual difficulties; chronic pain; weight or eating problems; gastrointestinal problems

Among users of VA health care, medical record data indicates that diagnoses of posttraumatic stress disorder (PTSD) and other anxiety disorders, depression and other mood disorders, and substance use disorders are most frequently associated with MST.

Fortunately, people can recover from experiences of trauma, and the VA has services to help veterans do this.

Services Available to Veterans

All veterans seen in VA health care are asked whether they experienced MST, and all treatment for physical and mental health conditions related to experiences of MST is free for both men and women.

Every VA healthcare facility has a designated MST coordinator who serves as a contact person for MST-related issues. This person can help veterans find and access VA services and programs. He or she may also be aware of state and federal benefits and community resources that may be helpful.

Every VA healthcare facility has providers knowledgeable about treatment for the aftereffects of MST. Many have specialized outpatient mental health services focusing on sexual trauma. Vet Centers also have specially trained sexual trauma counselors.

Nationwide, there are programs that offer specialized sexual trauma treatment in residential or inpatient settings. These are programs for veterans who need more intense treatment and support.

To accommodate veterans who do not feel comfortable in mixed-gender treatment settings, some facilities have separate programs for men and women. All residential and inpatient MST programs have separate sleeping areas for men and women.

To receive free, confidential treatment for mental and physical health conditions related to MST, veterans do not need to be service connected (have a VA disability rating). Veterans may be able to receive this benefit even if they are not eligible for other VA care. Veterans do not need to have reported the incident(s) when they happened or have other documentation that they occurred.

INTIMACY ISSUES

At first, many service members feel disconnected or detached from their partner and/or family. You may be unable to tell your family about what happened. You may not want to scare them by speaking about the war. Or maybe you think that no one will understand. You also may find it's hard to express positive feelings. This can make loved ones feel like they did something wrong or are not wanted anymore. Sexual closeness may also be awkward for a while. Remember, it takes time to feel close again. Intimacy is a combination of emotional *and* physical togetherness. It is not easily reestablished after stressful separations creating an emotional disconnect.

Partners may also experience high or low sexual interest causing disappointment, friction, or a sense of rejection. In due time, this may pass, but present concerns may include hoping one is still loved, dealing with rumors or concern about faithfulness, concern about medications that can affect desire and performance, and unexpected fatigue and alterations in sleep cycles.

What Are the Treatment Options?

It is essential to get proper counseling whether you are the victim of sexual abuse or are experiencing emotional issues that are affecting your sex life.

While military sexual trauma can be a very difficult experience, recovery is possible. Treatment can help improve your quality of life by focusing on strategies for managing emotions and memories or, for veterans who are ready, involve actually talking about their MST experiences in depth.

How Can Family and Friends Assist?

Many veterans who are the victims of sexual trauma do not tell family and friends. It is important to understand why revealing something like this can be so difficult. Victims in the military cannot leave their jobs, and they may have to continue working alongside their attacker, often in very dangerous circumstances. Until recently there were no real channels for making confidential complaints about MST, so many victims remained silent lest they affect their chances of promotion. Equally important, even when a formal complaint was made, the perpetrator more often than not simply received a slap on the wrist. That is why many victims remain silent and need the love and understanding that families and friends can provide.

For more information, veterans can speak with their existing VA healthcare provider, contact the MST coordinator at their nearest VA Medical Center, or contact their local Vet Center. A list of VA and Vet Center facilities can be found online by using the VA Facility Locator or Vet Center Locator. Veterans should feel free to ask to meet with a clinician of a particular gender if it would make them feel more comfortable. Veterans can also call the VA's general information hotline at 1-800-827-1000.

Other Resources

MakeTheConnection.net. Visit this site to view stories of veterans who have overcome military sexual trauma. MakeTheConnection.net is a one-stop resource where veterans and their families and friends can privately explore information on mental health issues, hear fellow veterans and their families share their stories of resilience, and easily find and access the support and resources they need.

AfterDeployment.org provides a program designed to provide support to service members who are healing after having experienced
sexual trauma.

MyDuty.mil. If you are an active-duty service member and have
been a victim of MST (or know someone who has), MyDuty.mil
provides information and guidance on your reporting options and
rights.

DOMESTIC VIOLENCE AND STALKING

On the evening of November 8, 2001, Ana Melina Kilic was at her job in
a hair-accessory shop in Harborplace, Baltimore's showpiece downtown
tourist and shopping area. At about 7 p.m., her ex-husband, Imamali Kilic,
appeared in the shop with a butcher knife. Ana Kilic fled, screaming, into
the corridor. Imamali Kilic overtook her, grabbed her, and, according to
more than 20 horrified witnesses, stabbed her again and again. He kept
stabbing even when about a dozen onlookers, one of them wielding a
baseball bat from a nearby sports store, rushed to Ana Kilic's rescue. They
eventually subdued him, but not in time to save his victim's life. An autopsy
later determined that the 28-year-old Ana Kilic had been stabbed or slashed
29 separate times. Imamali Kilic was arrested at the scene and charged with
murder. Not quite four months later, he hung himself in his cell at the
Baltimore City Jail, where he was awaiting trial. After surviving for a few
days on a respirator, he died on March 1, 2002.

The killing of Ana Kilic did not come unexpectedly out of the blue
or without any efforts to prevent it—quite the opposite. In August 2001, a
day after an earlier confrontation in her shop, she went to court to ask for
a restraining order against her husband, whose own workplace was in the
same Harborplace pavilion, one floor below. Her petition alleged that he
had raped her on two occasions and, in their encounter the previous day,
had threatened her with violence. The court granted a week-long restraining order, but then dismissed the case when Ana Kilic did not come back
to ask for its extension. About that time, the couple's divorce became final.

A little more than a month later, Ana Kilic complained to Baltimore
police that her ex-husband had abducted her, taken her to New Jersey, and
raped her again. Subsequently, according to police and court records, he
made threatening calls to her home, warning that he would kill her and
"cut off her arms and legs." He came to the shop and repeated the threats
to her face, Ana Kilic told police. Arrested on charges of harassment and

telephone misuse, Imamali Kilic spent a month in jail awaiting trial, then pleaded guilty to both offenses. Judge Paul A. Smith of the Baltimore Circuit Court sentenced him to three years of probation. The judge also ordered him to attend a program at a battered women's shelter and to have no contact with his ex-wife. With that, Imamali Kilic was released from jail. One day later, Ana Kilic was murdered.

The Kilic tragedy and the events that foreshadowed it illustrate one component of workplace violence: violence by a domestic partner or arising from another personal relationship that then follows someone to work. Domestic violence is a pattern of behavior in which one intimate partner uses physical violence; coercion; threats; intimidation; isolation; and emotional, sexual, or economic abuse to control the other partner in a relationship (American Bar Association Commission on Domestic Violence, *A Guide for Employees: Domestic Violence in the Workplace* [Washington, DC: 1999], 11).

Stalking or other harassing behavior is often an integral part of domestic violence and is as prevalent in the military as it is in civilian life. According to a study by the University of Iowa Injury Prevention Research Center (*Workplace Violence: A Report to the Nation* [Iowa City: February 2001], 12), 5 percent of workplace homicides (i.e., about one-third of homicides not associated with a robbery or other "stranger" crime) fall into this category.

Homicides, of course, represent a tiny fraction of workplace incidents related to domestic violence. Far more frequent are cases of stalking, threats, and harassment. Often those acts are criminal offenses in their own right; however, even when harassment may not meet the legal standard for criminal penalties, it can be frightening and disruptive not just for the person who is the target, but for coworkers, as well.

Frequently, employers are hesitant about involving themselves with an employee's personal relationships. Privacy is a legitimate concern, and finding the proper boundary between private and business affairs can be a difficult and sensitive matter. But domestic violence and stalking that come through the workplace door appropriately become the employer's concern too. Just as a business takes responsibility for protecting its workers from assaults or robberies by outsiders, it is also responsible for protecting them against stalking or other possible crimes by domestic partners.

Studies have shown that the most common stalking situations that law enforcement has to deal with are those based upon some type of personal relationship, with women primarily being victimized by males as a result of this behavior. However, in a smaller percentage of cases, both men and women can be stalked and harassed by casual acquaintances or strangers.

Observable Behavior That May Suggest Possible Victimization

- Tardiness or unexplained absences
- Frequent, and often unplanned, use of leave time
- Anxiety
- Lack of concentration
- Change in job performance
- A tendency to remain isolated from coworkers or reluctance to participate in social events
- Discomfort when communicating with others
- Disruptive phone calls or e-mail
- Sudden or unexplained requests to be moved from public locations in the workplace, such as sales or reception areas
- Frequent financial problems indicating lack of access to money
- Unexplained bruises or injuries
- Noticeable change in use of makeup (to cover up injuries)
- Inappropriate clothes (e.g., sunglasses worn inside the building, turtleneck worn in the summer)
- Disruptive visits from current or former intimate partner
- Sudden changes of address or reluctance to divulge where one is staying
- Acting uncharacteristically moody, depressed, or distracted
- In the process of ending an intimate relationship; breakup seems to cause the employee undue anxiety
- Court appearances
- Being the victim of vandalism or threats

Domestic violence and workplace violence are also related in another way: as noted earlier in this report, the evolution of domestic violence during the last several decades as a specific legal, social, and law enforcement issue can provide a model for similarly identifying and developing responses to violence in the workplace.

A particular concern when domestic and workplace violence intersects is the possibility that the victim, not the offender, will end up being punished. All too frequently, when an employee is being stalked, harassed, or threatened at work, an employer will decide that the quickest and easiest solution is to kick the problem out the door and fire the employee, rather than look for ways to protect her and her coworkers. Though common, especially when low-status, low-paying jobs are involved, this practice raises obvious ethical questions—and possibly issues of legal liability, as well. As with any other threat, the first requirement for protecting employees from domestic violence and/or stalking at the workplace is finding out that the threat exists. This can be particularly difficult in domestic abuse cases, where abuse victims often remain silent out of shame, embarrassment, a sense of helplessness, and fear.

Just as a supportive workplace climate makes employees feel safe in reporting other threats, an environment of trust and respect will make it easier for someone fearing domestic violence or stalking to tell an employer and seek assistance or protection. Perhaps more than with any other risk, employees facing domestic threats may tend to confide most easily in coworkers, rather than supervisors, managers, or a company's security force. It is also coworkers who are most likely to sense that someone they work with may be at risk from an abusive relationship, even if the person doesn't say anything explicitly.

Employers need to be careful about violating privacy or asking employees to break a coworker's confidence, but it is entirely reasonable and justifiable to encourage disclosure when others in the workplace may also be in danger. Beyond trying to create and maintain a generally supportive workplace atmosphere, employers can provide specific training to help the workforce to be more aware and sensitive to signs of possible domestic abuse. Training can also include teaching ways to persuade a reluctant coworker to tell supervisors and accept help an employer may be able to offer. Although domestic violence and stalking are largely thought of as violence against women and thus as a "woman's problem," training and awareness programs should be directed at all employees, men and women alike.

For employees involved in security or who will take part in the threat assessment and response, an employer can offer additional training focusing on how best to deal with domestic abuse victims. The same or similar training should be provided to anyone working with victims in a company's Employment Assistance Program. Both in training efforts and in providing help to at-risk workers, employers should draw on outside resources as well as their own: law enforcement, women's law and antiviolence advocacy groups, and social service agencies, for example.

When an employer becomes aware that an employee is being stalked, harassed, threatened, or abused and that the risk has or may come into the workplace, the threat should be subjected to the same evaluation procedure as any other violent threat, to assess the likelihood of violence and determine the best means of intervention. In almost all cases, employers should advise police of the circumstances, risk of violence, and possible criminal violations (e.g., of harassment or stalking laws) and involve law enforcement professionals in assessing and managing the threat. During and after the assessment, someone—from security, human resources, or a supervisor—should be responsible for keeping in close touch with the abuse victim, not only to help protect his/her safety and meet any needs that arise, but also to make sure of receiving any relevant information about the abuser (whom the victim, presumably, will know better than anyone else in her workplace).

Other Steps

- Referring the employee for emotional, legal, or financial counseling, either through the company's own employee assistance structure or from outside practitioners (e.g., a battered women's shelter or similar programs).
- Ascertaining if the employee has sought or obtained a protective "stay-away" court order against an abusive partner or other harasser.
- Adopting policies that will allow an abused worker time off for purposes such as going to court to seek a restraining order or appearing to testify at a criminal trial.
- Reviewing the employee's workspace and modifying it, if necessary, to make sure that a possible assailant cannot get there.
- Acting consistently with the employee's privacy rights and wishes and taking measures to inform other employees (e.g., security guards, secretaries, receptionists, and telephone operators) so they can block an abuser's calls or make sure he is kept out of the workplace.

Employers may consider other actions, as well. One option would be to help an employee obtain a restraining order (or obtain one on its own to keep a harasser off company property). Another would be to extend protective measures away from the worksite, looking at other places a worker may regularly go, such as a school or daycare facility where her children are enrolled, for example, and suggesting precautions that could be taken.

Actions That Reduce the Risk of Harm or Future Violence

Seek an evaluation and advice from a qualified mental health professional or crisis-intervention specialist if there are any critical risk factors.

Review and familiarize yourself with the material on the Internet that pertains to crisis intervention.

Seek counseling or therapy from a qualified mental health professional for any emotional problems or difficulties associated with angry or violent behavior.

Evaluate any alcohol and other drug use and treat as recommended by a qualified professional.

Encourage a medical evaluation and treatment for any mental illness or other medical condition requiring medication or medical treatment.

If appropriate, consider enrolling and participating in an educational or skills training group that will improve communication and interpersonal skills.

Develop a plan that will minimize and limit all communication that usually leads to conflict, aggression, or violence and take steps to resolve problems calmly.

Establish a plan that supports communication that does not increase the risk of violence and will support actions that reduce the risk of violence.

Ensure your own safety, and provide for your basic emotional and physical needs while allowing the other person to do the same.

If there is physical or sexual abuse, seek advice and further investigation from law enforcement or an attorney who has experience dealing with interpersonal violence, especially when violent or homicidal threats have been made. If appropriate, keep records of all contact, conversations, and threats made by the person including dates, times, and witnesses.

If appropriate, enroll in a personal safety and self-defense course. Information regarding these courses can usually be obtained through local telephone crisis services, healthcare facilities, or through the police or sheriff's department.

DEPRESSION

There are many emotional and psychological reactions that victims of rape and sexual assault can experience. One of the most common of these is depression.

The term "depression" can be confusing since many of the symptoms are experienced by people as normal reactions to events in their life. At some point or another, everyone feels sad or "blue," and these feelings are perfectly normal, especially during difficult times. But this also means that recognizing depression can be difficult since the symptoms can easily be attributed to other causes.

Therefore, if you experience five or more symptoms of depression over the course of two weeks, you should consider talking to a medical professional about what you are experiencing.

The symptoms for depression include:

prolonged sadness or unexplained crying spells;
change in appetite with significant weight loss (without dieting) or weight gain;
loss of energy, persistent fatigue, or lethargy;
significant change in sleep patterns (insomnia, sleeping too much, fitful sleep, etc.);
loss of interest and pleasure in activities previously enjoyed, social withdrawal;
feelings of worthlessness, hopelessness, or inappropriate guilt;
pessimism or indifference;
unexplained aches and pains (headaches, stomachaches);
inability to concentrate, indecisiveness;
irritability, worry, anger, agitation, or anxiety; and
recurring thoughts of death or suicide.

If you are having suicidal thoughts, don't wait to get help. Call the Telephone Helpline at 877-995-5247 (the phone number is the same inside the United States or via the DSN), or the National Veterans Suicide Prevention Lifeline at 800-273-TALK (8255) at any time (veterans press 1).

Depression can affect anyone of any age, gender, race, ethnicity, or religion. Depression is not a sign of weakness, and it is not something that someone can simply "snap out of."

SELF-HARM/SELF-INJURY

Deliberate self-harm, or self-injury, is when a person inflicts physical harm on himself or herself, usually in secret. Some victims of sexual assault may use self-harm to cope with the difficult or painful feelings, but it is only a temporary relief, not a healthy way to deal with the trauma of sexual assault. Self-harm can cause permanent damage to the body, as well as additional psychological problems that hinder the healing process, such as guilt, depression, low self-esteem, or self-hatred, along with a tendency toward isolation.

Note: Deliberate self-harm is not necessarily inflicted with suicidal intent, and engaging in self-harm does not necessarily mean that someone wants to die.

What to Watch For

For sexual assault victims, self-injury may:

provide a way to express difficult or hidden feelings. It's common for victims to feel numb or empty as a result of sexual assault;

provide a temporary sense of feeling again, as well as a way to express anger, sadness, grief, or emotional pain;

provide a way of communicating to others that support is needed;

provide a distraction from emotional pain;

provide self-punishment for what they believe they deserve;

provide proof that they are not invisible; and

provide a feeling of control. It's not uncommon to feel that self-harm is the only way to have a sense of control over life, feelings, body, especially if other things in life are out of control.

Some common methods of self-harm include:

cutting;
burning;
biting;
hitting the body;
pulling out hair;
scratching and picking at sores on skin;
eating disorders; and
substance abuse.

Helping Someone You Know

Friends and family of sexual assault victims may be among the first to recognize the signs of self-injury. It may be helpful for a survivor to share their experiences and concerns with a qualified service provider who can help him or her find a healthier, positive alternative to alleviate the pain from sexual assault, such as a counselor or psychologist. It may be helpful for the survivor to have the help and support of a loved one while finding a counselor. If the survivor feels that talking with someone is too overwhelming, you can urge him or her to write down the problem.

Alternatives

The following are alternatives to self-harm that may help you until you are able to meet with a professional.

Recognize the choices you have NOW; ask yourself what YOU need.
Choose to put off self-harm for specific amounts of time until a professional can be contacted (e.g., 15-minute increments).
Count down to relaxation (10 . . . 9 . . . 8 . . . 7 . . .); start meditation exercises; pay attention to your breathing and the rhythmic motions of your body.
Write in a diary or journal.
Make a list of people you can call for support; connect with others (group, one-on-one).
Plan something new and exciting to do with friends.
Take up a craft (needlework, quilting, painting, etc.).
Play video games, listen to the radio, or watch television as a distraction.

It is important to eat well, exercise, and be kind to oneself. While not a solution in itself, doing all these things can contribute to increased mood stability and a general better sense of well-being that will provide a greater sense of happiness on the inside and outside.

Get Help

If you or someone you know is contemplating suicide, call 911 immediately (in the United States). If there's no one in your life that you feel comfortable talking to about your suicidal thoughts, call the National Veterans Suicide Prevention Lifeline at 800-273-TALK (8255) at any time (veterans press 1).

EATING DISORDERS

Eating disorders are complex conditions that arise from a combination of long-standing emotional, psychological, interpersonal, and social issues. People with eating disorders often use food and the control of food as an attempt to deal with or compensate for feelings and emotions that may otherwise seem overwhelming.

Causes

Sexual assault or abuse can have an effect on the victim's perceived body image and affect their eating habits. For some victims, self-starvation, bingeing, and purging may begin as a way to cope with the trauma of the assault or to feel in control of a certain aspect of their lives. But, ultimately, the damage caused by eating disorders can worsen their physical and emotional health as well as their self-esteem.

Factors stemming from sexual abuse that may result in an eating disorder include:

low self-esteem;
feelings of inadequacy or lack of control in life;
depression, anxiety, anger, or loneliness; and
difficulty expressing emotions and feelings.

Help a Friend

While each situation is different, there are some general guidelines to consider if you know or suspect someone you love is suffering from an eating disorder:

Set aside time to meet with your loved one to discuss your concerns openly, honestly, and in a supportive way.
Stay away from accusatory statements; use words like "I feel," "I wish," "I hope."
Remind your loved one that you care and want to support him or her in any way you can.

Anorexia Nervosa

A serious, potentially life-threatening eating disorder characterized by self-starvation and excessive weight loss. The four primary symptoms are resistance to maintaining body weight, intense fear of weight gain, denial of the seriousness of low body weight, and loss of menstrual periods in girls/women.

Warning signs include: dramatic weight loss, preoccupation with weight and food, refusal to eat certain foods, frequent comments about feeling "fat," anxiety about gaining weight, denial of hunger, development of food rituals, consistent excuses to avoid mealtimes, rigid exercise regimen despite weather or fatigue, and withdrawal from usual friends and activities.

Health consequences include: abnormally slow heart rate and low blood pressure, reduction of bone density (osteoporosis), muscle loss and weakness, severe dehydration, fainting, and dry hair and skin.

Binge Eating Disorder

Eating disorder characterized by recurrent binge eating without the regular use of compensatory measures to counter the binge eating.

The four primary symptoms are frequent episodes of eating large quantities of food in short periods of time, feeling out of control over eating behavior, feeling ashamed or disgusted by the behavior, and eating when not hungry and eating in secret.

Health consequences include: high blood pressure, high cholesterol levels, heart disease, diabetes mellitus, and gallbladder disease.

Bulimia Nervosa

Serious, potentially life-threatening eating disorder characterized by a cycle of bingeing and compensatory behaviors such as self-induced vomiting designed to undo or compensate for the effects of binge eating.

The three primary symptoms are regular intake of large amounts of food accompanied by a sense of loss of control over eating behavior; regular use of inappropriate compensatory behavior such as self-induced vomiting or laxative abuse or fasting; and extreme concern with body weight and shape.

Warning signs include disappearance of large amounts of food in short periods of time, frequent trips to the bathroom after meals, rigid exercise regimen despite weather or fatigue, unusual swelling of cheeks or jaw area, calluses on the back of the hands and knuckles, discoloration or staining of teeth, and withdrawal from usual friends and activities.

Health consequences include electrolyte imbalances that can lead to irregular heartbeats and possibly heart failure, inflammation and possible rupture of the esophagus from frequent vomiting, tooth decay and staining from stomach acids released during vomiting, chronic irregular bowel movements and constipation as a result of laxative abuse, and gastric rupture.

Get Help

The most effective and long-lasting treatment for eating disorders is a form of therapy. Each treatment will vary according to the patient's particular issues, needs, and strengths.

> Psychological counseling—a licensed health professional addresses both the eating disorder symptoms and the underlying forces that contributed (in this case, sexual assault)
> Outpatient therapy—support groups, nutritional counseling, and/or psychiatric medications under careful supervision
> Hospital-based care—necessary when an eating disorder has led to physical problems that may be life-threatening, or when it is associated with severe psychological or behavioral problems

Additional Resources

National Eating Disorders Association (www.nationaleatingdisorders.org)
The Academy of Nutrition and Dietetics (www.eatright.org)
BodyImageHealth.org (http://bodyimagehealth.org)
Eating Disorders Anonymous (www.eatingdisordersanonymous.org)

POST-TRAUMATIC STRESS DISORDER

Survivors of sexual assault may experience severe feelings of anxiety, stress, or fear known as post-traumatic stress disorder (PTSD) as a direct result of the assault. While it is natural to have some of these symptoms after a traumatic event, if they last more than a few weeks and become an ongoing problem, it might be PTSD. The symptoms of PTSD are grouped into three categories.

Re-experiencing Symptoms

May cause problems in everyday routine.

> Flashbacks—reliving the trauma over and over, including physical symptoms like racing heart or sweating

Bad dreams—subconscious memories of the event

Frightening thoughts—can be triggered by specific words, objects, or situations

Avoidance Symptoms

May cause the survivor to change his or her personal routine.

Avoiding specific places, events, or objects
Feeling emotionally numb
Feeling strong guilt, depression, or worry
Losing interest in activities that were enjoyable in the past
Having trouble remembering the frightening event

Hyperarousal Symptoms

May cause difficulty in completing daily tasks, such as sleeping, eating, or concentrating.

Being easily startled
Feeling tense or "on edge"
Having difficulty sleeping, and/or having angry outbursts

Children and teens can have extreme reactions to trauma, and their symptoms may not be the same as adults. Symptoms may include:

bedwetting;
inability to talk;
acting out the assault during playtime; and
being unusually clingy with a parent or other trusted adult.

To be diagnosed with PTSD, a doctor who has experience helping people with mental illnesses, such as a psychiatrist or psychologist, must speak with the survivor.

Treatment

For more information, visit: National Center for PTSD: www.ptsd.va.gov.

If you know or suspect someone you love is suffering from PTSD:

Offer emotional support, understanding, patience, and encouragement.

Learn about PTSD, including available recovery resources, so you can understand what your loved one is experiencing and help him or her seek help.

SLEEP DISTURBANCES

Many survivors of sexual assault suffer from depression and/or PTSD. As a result, they may also experience sleep disturbances and disorders. Sleep can be difficult for trauma victims, as they may not feel secure and unthreatened.

Nightmares

Nightmares can result when an assault is replayed mentally and when there is a fear that it will reoccur. Nightmares typically involve feelings and emotions felt at the time of the assault or abuse, or immediately following, and can cause difficulty in falling and staying asleep. Individuals may report multiple nightmares within a given night, often with a recurrent theme. Nightmares usually end with an awakening of full alertness and lingering sense of fear or anxiety.

If nighttime awakenings are frequent, or if the individual avoids sleeping because of fear that a nightmare will occur, the individual may experience the following:

excessive sleepiness;
poor concentration;
depression;
anxiety; and
irritability.

This form of sleep disturbance is not diagnosed if the nightmares occur exclusively during the course of another mental disorder or are due to the direct effects of substance abuse (alcohol, drugs, or medication) or a general medical condition.

Insomnia

Insomnia can be described as difficulty falling asleep, difficulty staying asleep, or waking up too early. These periods of restlessness can last a few nights or become chronic and last several months, or even years.

Insomnia can be caused by:

life events that cause physical, emotional, or mental pain;
anxiety about falling asleep, stress;
medication (a possible side effect);
environmental noise or extreme temperature changes; and
herbs, caffeine, alcohol, or other substances.

Physicians and therapists may suggest trying medication or behavioral techniques to improve sleep, such as relaxation therapy, sleep restriction, and reconditioning. For more information, contact your physician.

Sleep Terror

Sleep terror disorder occurs with repeated abrupt awakenings from sleep, usually beginning with a panicky scream or cry. During an episode, the individual is going through behavioral manifestations of intense fear and is difficult to awaken or comfort. After finally waking, the individual has no recollection of the event except perhaps a single image.

During a sleep terror, the individual may actively resist being held or touched or even demonstrate more elaborate activity (swinging, punching, fleeing). These behaviors appear to represent self-protection from a threat and may result in physical injury.

Sleep terror disorder may occur with an increased frequency in individuals with PTSD and generalized anxiety disorder. Many individuals suffer from isolated episodes of sleep terrors at some time in their lives. The distinction between individual episodes and sleep terror disorder lies in the repeated occurrence and potential for self-injury. Eating well, exercising, and getting help for sleep disorders can be useful in treating them. Increased mood stability and a general better sense of well-being will provide a greater sense of ease, and will make nighttime sleep a safe space once again.

SUBSTANCE ABUSE

Victims of rape or sexual assault may turn to alcohol or other substances in an attempt to relieve their emotional suffering. In the United States, victims of sexual assault report higher levels of psychological distress and the consumption of alcohol than non-victims, in part to self-medicate. Some victims use substances to cope with the reality of what happened to them or to cope with the symptoms of PTSD, a common reaction to an extreme situation like sexual assault. However, it is not a healthy way to deal with the trauma of sexual assault and can cause additional problems, such as addiction or dependence, which hinder the healing process.

A survivor of sexual assault or sexual abuse in his or her childhood may abuse drugs to help "numb out" and push away the painful memories of sexual violence. Victims may also turn to drugs instead of true recovery resources, such as counseling. Some possible explanations for this are that they may not think that friends or family will understand them, they may not know where to access recovery resources, or they may be embarrassed to talk about what happened.

Friends and family of sexual assault victims may be among the first to recognize the signs of substance abuse. Early recognition increases chances for successful treatment. Warning signs include:

> giving up past activities or hobbies;
> spending time with new friends who may be a negative influence;
> declining grades or performance at work;
> aggressiveness, irritability;
> forgetfulness;
> disappearing money or valuables from family and friends;
> lying;
> depression or hopelessness;
> avoiding friends and family;
> drinking and driving or getting in trouble with the law; and
> suspension from school or work.

When compared to non-victims, rape survivors are 3.4 times more likely to use marijuana, 6 times more likely to use cocaine, and 10 times more likely to use other major drugs.

Finding Treatment

Most substance abusers believe they can stop using drugs on their own, but many who try to stop do not succeed. Research shows that long-term drug use alters brain function and strengthens compulsions to use drugs. This craving continues even after the drug use stops. Because of these ongoing cravings, the most important component of treatment is preventing relapse.

It may be helpful for a survivor to share their experiences and concerns with a qualified service provider (e.g., a counselor or psychologist). A general physician can suggest community resources as well as prescribe medications to control cravings and withdrawal symptoms while the user seeks further help.

If you feel you are suffering from substance abuse:

Reach out to a trusted friend or family member and ask for help.

Contact the free Substance Abuse Treatment Referral Helpline, 1-800-662-HELP (4357).

Contact a doctor.

Contact your doctor immediately if you are suffering from a cough that won't go away, fever, continuing feelings of depression, jaundice, mild tremors, leg swelling, or increased abdominal girth.

Call 911 (inside the United States) or go to a hospital's emergency department immediately if you are suffering from severe abdominal pain, chest pain, rapid heartbeat, severe tremors, numbness, or suicidal thoughts.

Help Someone You Know

If someone you know is suffering from substance abuse:

Contact the free Substance Abuse Treatment Referral Helpline, 1-800-662-HELP (4357), for support and advice on helping your loved one.

Do not "cover up" for your loved one. It is important that he or she gets the help that he or she deserves.

It is also best to speak to your loved one shortly after a substance-related problem has occurred (like a serious family argument or accident).

Gather information in advance about treatment options in your community. If the person is willing to get help, seek help immediately and offer to go with him or her for support.

Additional Resources

Alcoholics Anonymous (www.aa.org)

United States Department of Health and Human Services Substance Abuse and Mental Health Services Administration (www.samhsa. gov)

Substance Abuse Treatment Facility Locator (http://findtreatment. samhsa.gov)

Toll-Free Substance Abuse Treatment Referral Helpline, 1-800-662-HELP (1-800-662-4357)

The National Institute on Drug Abuse (NIDA) (www.drugabuse.gov)

SUICIDE

Many of the devastating emotional and psychological reactions that victims of rape and sexual assault can experience can eventually lead to thoughts of suicide. There are also many military-specific factors that may increase the risk of suicidal thoughts. These factors include: frequent deployments, deployments to hostile environments, exposure to extreme stress, physical or sexual assault while in the service (not limited to women), length of deployments, or service-related injury.

If you are currently thinking about suicide, please reach out for help. Warning signs include:

talking about or threatening to hurt or kill oneself;

looking for ways to kill oneself by seeking access to firearms, available pills, or other means;

talking or writing about death more than usual;

feeling hopeless;

feeling rage or uncontrolled anger or seeking revenge;

acting reckless or engaging in risky activities—seemingly without thinking;

feeling trapped—like there's no way out;

increasing alcohol or drug use;

withdrawing from friends, family, and society;

feeling anxious, agitated, or unable to sleep or sleeping all the time;

experiencing dramatic mood changes;

seeing no reason for living or having no sense of purpose in life;

giving away treasured possessions;

preparing for death, which might mean making a will and/or taking care of tax and/or legal issues;

talking about suicide directly; and

talking about suicide indirectly.

Comments like "Things would be better if I weren't here," "I just wish I could die," and "I just want to go to sleep and never wake up" can be indirect clues that someone is thinking about suicide.

If you are having suicidal thoughts:

Call 911 (inside the United States) or go to the hospital.

If you have already taken steps to harm yourself or feel that you can't stop yourself from committing suicide, call 911 (inside the United States) or go to the emergency room. Tell the person on the phone or the front desk at the emergency room that you are suicidal.

Call the National Veterans Suicide Prevention Lifeline at 800-273-TALK (8255) at any time (veterans press 1). Counselors there can talk to you about ways to resolve the situation that has made you think about suicide and can connect you with resources to help you.

Reach out to friends, family, or someone you trust. Let them know that you are going through a rough time.

Find a doctor, counselor, or therapist who can help you figure out how to resolve your situation.

Get rid of the means. If you have been thinking about committing suicide and you have obtained the means to commit suicide, please get rid of it. If you have a gun, give it to someone you trust. If you have pills, flush them down the toilet.

If someone you know is having suicidal thoughts:

Contact Safe Helpline or the National Veterans Suicide Prevention Lifeline at any time. You can call this number even if you are not suicidal. The counselor will be able to work with you to help you help the person you're concerned about.

Take his/her words seriously.

Be willing to listen and allow him or her to express his or her feelings freely.

Get involved, become available, and show interest and support.

Don't judge.

Don't act shocked—this will put distance between you.

Don't be sworn to secrecy—seek support.

Don't debate whether suicide is right or wrong, and don't lecture on the value of life.

Avoid comments that dismiss the suicidal person, like:

"Things can't be that bad."

"You're just talking about suicide."

"You wouldn't really do that."

Asking about suicidal thoughts will not make someone commit suicide:

Ask, "Are you thinking about suicide?"

Ask if they have a plan for how they would commit suicide and the means to carry out the plan.

If they are planning to commit suicide and they have a plan and the means to carry out the plan, you should get help for this person as quickly as possible—call 911 (inside the United States) or take them to the emergency room.

Try not to leave them alone.

You can also remove the means to commit suicide, but only if you can do it safely.

If they are not planning to commit suicide immediately, offer support.

Work with the person to figure out alternative ways to resolve the situation.

You can also offer practical help by giving them hotline numbers, finding support groups, or giving them rides to appointments.

Follow up by calling or visiting to see how they're doing and whether or not things are improving.

Additional Resources

National Suicide Prevention Lifeline (www.suicidepreventionlifeline. org)

National Suicide Prevention Lifeline—Veterans (http://veteranscrisisline.net)

Toll-Free National Suicide Prevention Lifeline: 800-273-TALK (8255), veterans press 1. For hearing and speech impaired with TTY equipment: 800-799-4TTY (4889)

5

CASE STUDIES

Jennifer Norris, U.S. Air Force

The STOP (Sexual Assault Training Oversight and Prevention) Act would establish an independent professional legal entity separate from the chain of command of the Department of Defense. Until very recently, sexual assault investigations were under the control of and conducted by the commander. The commander had the power to decide to pursue justice or not and to what level he elevated it. Leon Panetta, then secretary of defense (July 2011–February 2013), had recently declared that he was taking the power to investigate out of the hands of the commanders and giving it to an O-6 or higher in the chain of command. My initial reaction is that there is an automatic conflict of interest with that and that the investigation can still be stifled if kept within the chain of command. The STOP Act would help to provide a form of checks and balances and put the case in the hands of a professional so that the investigation is handled appropriately. It is imperative that these cases be handled effectively in order to prevent further emotional and physical harm to the victims of such crimes.

In my efforts to educate the public via mostly social media, my fellow advocacy peers and I have come across rape apologists. My initial reaction is that these vocal dissenters of justice are the perpetrators themselves, but after seeing so many various reactions to the topic, I am led to believe that there is a widespread misconception out there about the crime, the perpetrators, and the victims of sexual assault. For some reason, the white elephant in the room is that most claims of sexual assault are bogus reports. Today I was reminded by a fellow soldier (not the norm) that victims of rape claim rape to avoid charges of adultery. Who would know about that aside from the rapists and those unfortunate victims who happen to get caught up in this web of destruction? I never would have imagined this kind of response to a person who had the courage to report this crime. My day was somewhat planned until I woke up to this kind of mentality once again.

Instead of turning the other way and doing nothing, I decided to take this opportunity to educate others about the issue since there really is no arguing with idiots. At this point, it isn't about what the rape apologists have to say; it's about the truth. The truth is that most reports of sexual assault are not bogus reports. If there are any cases of bogus reports, they are definitely not the norm and don't even compare to the number of sexual assaults. By the DoD's own estimates there are roughly 3,192 sexual assaults reported each year in the military. These DoD estimates are staggering. Although Secretary Panetta estimates that the number is closer to 19,000 a year, most of them go unreported. And for those who have been victims of sexual assault or rape in the military, you understand clearly why one would be hesitant to report. It has devastating effects on your career, and in some cases reporting this crime is a career ender.

Although I pressed charges against two of the four perpetrators I crossed paths with within the first two years of my career, justice was still not served. I thought at the time that justice was served, but after seeing how things played out and learning more about the issue, I see that my case clearly falls into the typical way that sexual assault investigations are handled in the military. The threshold for punishment is one of pity for the perpetrator because of how the report might affect their career, and therefore they are not dealt the punishment that fits the crime. I must preface by stating that my commander handled the situation pretty well. Unfortunately, this is not the norm. I have read countless stories about military rape victims who have sought justice only to be met with disbelief. In addition, they are treated like the enemy afterward, and their lives become a living hell. Not only are they forced to work with their rapist, but they are also forced psychologically to handle a situation that no one would wish on their worst enemy. Imagine the psychological trauma that results from getting raped by a fellow soldier and then having to work with or for that individual the next day.

In my case, one of the men who was sexually assaulting me was my NCOIC (noncommissioned officer in charge). He was my boss, and therefore he had the power to tell me what to do and when to do it. I was an E-4, and he was an E-7. He had the power to make me a "warehouse manager" in an effort to isolate me so that he could prey on me when we were alone. If he told me to work in the warehouse that day, then I worked in the warehouse. If he told me to do anything, I had to do it because otherwise it was "disobeying a direct order" or "disrespect to an NCO." I knew that if I did not comply with him he could affect the outcome of my promotions, temporary duty assignments, work responsibilities, and general overall health. I was totally enslaved to this man, because I didn't want to risk the harm that came from reporting a sexual predator to the chain of command. Eventually, I didn't have a choice but to report, but it was not until after I was completely broken.

I went from "superior performer" to I don't give a crap. I went from I want to retire with the military to I want out of here as soon as I can. I went from being happy and energetic to being totally sad and completely wiped out emotionally. I never imagined in a million years how negatively this would affect my psyche. I now understood why it is illegal and considered a crime to touch another person's body; force yourself on another person; and/or make derogatory, sexual, belittling comments to another human being. I felt like my hard work and efforts meant nothing. I felt like I existed mainly for the purpose of the perpetrator's pleasure. I felt like no matter how hard I worked or how much I learned, none of it mattered. It was like banging my head against a brick wall. Others noticed how hard I worked, but the one person that controlled my career just happened to be a sexual predator.

For those who have been in the military, you understand how important the chain of command is. You also know that it is required that you report to your chain of command and attempt to resolve all issues at the lowest level possible. So what do you do when the person who is assaulting you is in your chain of command? I was approached by a senior NCO (E-7), outside my chain of command, who noticed that I had changed. He observed that I went from loving the military to not caring about anything. Being approached by this professional man who genuinely cared opened the floodgates. I finally broke down after months of attempting to handle the situation on my own with no success and told him what I had been dealing with on an almost daily basis. I was scared of my boss and no longer wanted to be subjected to his abuse and assaults.

My NCOIC purposefully set me up to be alone with him. And his predator ways escalated over time. After assigning me to tasks that put me in isolated positions, he would then show up and make his move. For example, I was the warehouse manager, so he assigned me to clean up and organize the warehouse. I welcomed the challenge of the work but dreaded the isolated moments that he took advantage of. He grabbed me, pushed himself on me, groped me, and tried to force me to be physical and intimate with him. I would fight him off and fight back. I professionally, assertively, and angrily told him not to touch me on numerous occasions.

He would not take no for an answer, and he would get angry with me after I rejected his advances. I was told that I should feel privileged that he was interested in me, that I was a bitch, and that he didn't want me anyway because I had small tits. So in addition to having my body violated, I was belittled and yelled at because I would not comply with his demands. This didn't happen once or twice. This happened on numerous occasions, if not daily at times. He escalated over time and became more angry, sneaky, manipulative, and forceful.

Had this man not had control over my career, I would have ceased the behavior sooner. But because I was trying to safeguard my career while politely (and not so politely) trying to reject his advances, I was always scared that he would abuse his power. He had the power to write me up, talk bad about me to leadership, and hinder promotion, in addition to taking advantage of me. I felt like I was under his complete control, and I worked every day trying to be perfect so that he could not use anything against me. Unfortunately, because he started to escalate and exhibit his behaviors in front of others, and no one said anything, it made me feel even more alone. I felt like I had nowhere to turn. I couldn't turn to my chain of command because he was in my chain of command. I did not even think about reporting the sexual assaults to my commander because the chain of command was so adamant about resolving issues at the lowest level possible. I also knew that if I reported this man for sexually assaulting me, my career would be over. And, in fact, it was.

Everyone in my chain of command was informed after I reported the assault. It was protocol to keep my supervisor, the chief, the officer-in-charge, and the perpetrator informed at all times. The commander knew everything, and it was his responsibility to keep the others in my chain of command informed with what was happening with one of their troops and the superintendent of maintenance. It was humiliating. And, instead of being supported through the process, I was judged, isolated, and basically run out. During the investigation, I was transferred out of the squadron. I agreed to the transfer because I could no longer handle being under the control of my NCOIC or in the same room with him. He had assaulted me on so many occasions that I was traumatized. I never knew when I was going to be put in a position where I had to fight him off. All I could think was, why can't I just come to work and work? Why do I have to deal with this? How do I make it stop?

The enacting of the STOP Act would provide me with a place to turn to, someone to advocate for me, and emotional help. Although my commander did the best he could to investigate the situation professionally, it put all parties involved in a difficult position. Most crimes are investigated by professionals who went to school to learn the art of investigation, forensics, and crime scene analysis. Commanders have a full-time job with their existing responsibilities, let alone investigating a sexual assault claim. At the time, there was no help for me. It was so unbelievable to me that I would get assaulted by another in uniform, prove this, and not be offered any kind of mental health services. As a matter of fact, I had to pay for these services out of pocket. And because I was having such a hard time coping with the assaults, coping with the long, drawn-out investigation process, and then coping with the retaliatory behavior by others in the squadron, I was devastated. I had no choice but to turn to a professional for help. I had never been exposed to this kind of behavior and quite frankly didn't even know what it was.

The STOP Act will hold perpetrators accountable, investigate the crimes, prosecute fairly, and provide checks and balances in the system. If this felony crime weren't so devastating, we would not have to create a special office to handle it, but it is. It is devastating not only to the victim but also to the squadron or unit as a whole. Morale was turned upside down after I reported the crime and the commander launched an investigation. It was a small unit, and the rumor mill started almost immediately. I was so ashamed of what had occurred that I was not interested in talking about the situation with anyone. Quite frankly, it was embarrassing and I wanted to put it behind me and move on. Unfortunately, others became fearful of me because they were not aware of what truly occurred. They were told that they had to be careful around me, that I was a troublemaker, and that I was a traitor. I never expected that response. I never expected that I would be betrayed in that way.

I would have preferred that the investigation be handled outside the squadron. I would have preferred that the case be handled discreetly. I would have preferred that I was offered mental health services. I would have preferred that both of us leave the squadron to prevent one or the other from talking about the circumstances in order to gain support. Removing the investigation from the chain of command would have changed the entire dynamic of the situation. The STOP Act emphasizes the importance of human rights, discourages criminal activity, encourages professionalism in the investigation, ensures the best possible outcome for a conviction that holds up, and prevents others from becoming a victim of that perpetrator as well. Criminal investigations are handled by the professionals in the civilian world; there is no reason why they shouldn't be handled by professionals in the military as well. The STOP Act would create a legal entity that specializes in the investigation and prosecution of these predators. The STOP Act would hold predators responsible and accountable for their criminal activity. Sexual assault and rape are not only felony crimes, but also human rights issues. The STOP Act will protect our defenders too.

★ ★ ★

Jennifer Norris currently works with the Military Rape Crisis Center as its Maine director.

M.T., FLORIDA

I joined the Air Force at age 18, in 1981. After basic and technical school I arrived at MacDill AFB. I was the first woman in my career field assigned to my shop and was not accepted at all.

My first roll call I was told that I would not be there long as I had no business invading this man's career field. I was told that I would be carried out in a body bag, commit suicide, go AWOL, or be put in a straightjacket before they were done with me.

Within a couple weeks I was attacked at the barracks (not raped) and suffered a head injury, which my attacker did in front of a group of people and never was charged. While in the hospital one of the supervisors started to befriend me. He built my trust up. At a party off base he followed me into a bathroom and raped me. I left and couldn't speak. Then in the middle of the night woke up in my barracks room to find him on top of me. I tried to say something but was told nothing will happen.

I became pregnant and was told I was to have an abortion. The supervisor was high-fiving the other supervisors when they found out because they can get rid of me. I don't believe in abortion and refused. I was dropped off every week at an abortion clinic off base and had to take a cab back to the base.

I had tools thrown at my head. I was harassed by everyone. Even the guy's wife would call or they would let her in the shop to yell and threaten me. I was sent to Eglin AFB psych unit. The doctor said I was normal and gave me a month to regroup and sent me back to the Hell awaiting me.

When I returned I was told to never wear maternity clothes. They tried to hide my pregnancy. My commanding officer (A WOMAN) asked me if she could send me to Europe TDY to get an abortion since I was 7 months pregnant. The harassing and threats continued. I had to move from the barracks to get some peace and got an apartment off base.

The wing commander asked me what was happening and I told him. He had me moved from the shop to another location. Nothing happened to anyone. I had the baby and was forced to give him up for adoption.

In 2007 we reunited and I found out the person who adopted him was a doctor at the base hospital and he and his wife were well aware of the situation and raised him to find me. The rapist is retired from the military and was never charged. I have lived in hell for the last 30+ years and just in the last few years can really speak about this. What is the military doing about the babies from MST? Not all of us believe in abortion. They are victims too.

J.R., U.S. AIR FORCE

After the assault I tried to appear fine when in reality I was falling apart inside. I didn't want my chain of command to know how and why I felt the way I did because I was judged, threatened, and expected to "suck it up," and my treatment and medications were used against me. I, too, was scheduled to go to Iraq in 2008 and had weaned off my medications so that I could do so. The VA was not willing to sign off on allowing me to deploy because they were afraid that I would have no support if something was to happen to me (they knew that I was trying to be strong but was ready to fall apart). I tried to fight them but in the end could not continue to hide the information from the military because of Q21 on my security clearance [Question 21 refers to mental health and requires a person to indicate whether he or she has had mental health issues]. Had I been supported from the get-go (1999) and allowed to get the help I needed without worrying about how it would affect my career, I could have gotten healthy a lot sooner. But, I was not supported at all. I felt I had to hide the information from my chain of command because it was used against me. I was judged as being "crazy," "on happy pills," "a national security risk," and "weak." This type of treatment only compounded the PTSD. I had no confidentiality if I did get help because everyone in the chain of command was informed. This also ties into why PTSD for MST survivors is so traumatic. The assaults themselves are very traumatic, personal, and shameful. We wouldn't see nearly as many PTSD claims as we do if it weren't for the continued abuse, judgment, and mistreatment by those in our chain of command. Instead, I would have still been serving my country while getting the help I needed to be the best soldier I could be.

ANONYMOUS, U.S. NAVY

On 16 November 2011 I was sitting at the ER at the Dayton VA and this male veteran approached me and asked me "to go out back and have sex with him." I said, "What?" He said, "Let's go out back and fuck." It brought back all my memories that I had hidden for so many years. I just got up and went back home and took an extra two diazepam. I was at the ER for my anxiety in the first place. It brought back so many memories of what happened to me when I was active duty and what happened to my children.

First, it was in June 5, 1982; I was 18, and at my first duty station in Roosevelt Roads, Puerto Rico. I lived in the Bundy Barracks and worked for the Navy Exchange (I ran a mini store at the main barracks). One night a friend named Sara asked me to go to the Seabee Club with her so I went one Saturday night. I remember we were talking to a couple of guys who had bought us a couple of cokes. I believe my coke was drugged because the next thing I remember was being at the bus stop alone the next morning waiting for a bus to be taken back to the Bundy Barracks. I do not remember what happened to Sara. As I was sitting there waiting for the bus I was having vivid memories of different men having sex with me. I did not know who they were or that they even knew me. I do not remember faces; all I could see in my mind was that there were several men. I have no clue as to whom or where I even was the night before or even how I got there.

The vivid memories I now have are of different men's penises in my mouth and in my vagina at different times throughout the night. I remember I was in such a daze in and out. My body was limp and I remember just lying there with no control over anything I did or was being done to me. I remember being dragged from one bed to another. I was completely out of it. I remember being at work the next Monday and this guy came in and told me everything that had happened. I did not realize that all that had happened. He told me that at least 25 different guys had sex with me.

I then went to the Naval Hospital and was told that if I was to report it that I would be put out of the Navy because it was destruction of government property and that it was my fault for being at the club. I also became pregnant and was diagnosed with herpes. I was also transferred from the department to MWR, because I "didn't fit in at the Naval Exchange" (NEX), as I was told.

Second around August of 1982 this one guy wanted to date me, and I was to have sex with him or he would get my friend in trouble (he was base police). I did not want it nor did I like it but I felt coerced into doing it. That had occurred a few times. I was transferred to the gym to work. I remember one day I was walking to work (I did not have a car) and these guys drove by me and yelled out, "Hey that is the chick we all fucked that one night" (my pregnancy was showing at this time).

Third time was between November and December 1982; the boss at the gym (★★★★★ ★★★★★) made me perform oral sex. I went to my sr. military officer and he told me that it was my word against the civilian's and no one would believe me, he told me that if I pursued it I would lose my career and asked how I would support my child and myself without the military. So I did not fight for my rights yet again. I then remember I was stationed at Gt. Lakes Naval Hospital, where I was the administration assistant to a Lt. who was the department head. He and I worked in the same small office. He made sexual advances toward me all the time. Told me I would have great evaluations and he could do a lot for me if I did certain sexually things. I kept telling him no. Because of all the above I have never been in a "real" relationship. I spent most of my time with my children watching movies, playing kids' games and doing kid things.

In September 1989, I received orders to Guantanamo Bay Cuba, and I had to leave my children behind until I received base housing. I worked with this sr. chief corpsman for over a year; he said he and his wife would take care of them. I paid them $1,500.00, took over clothes, and dropped my children and their clothes off with them. I came back 35 days later and picked up my kids to find them bruised and balled spots on their heads. Took them to a friend's house (Dental Tech Chief), I put my kids in the bath and they had bruises all over them and cigar burns on their bottoms, I then took my kids to the Naval Hospital to get pictures taken and contacted NIS.

There were reports done; my girls ages 6 and 3 were both sexually abused and my 2-year-old son was also. It took me 6 months to get my son to sleep on a bed and use a blanket and pillow. He would crawl in a corner and scream instead of going to sleep. November 1989 I started going to the Naval Hospital Mental Health Department and started medication for depression and anxiety, due to the sexual, physical, emotional abuse my children suffered. My children were beat with a wooden spoon; my youngest two had bald spots all over their heads. My middle daughter was made to eat like a dog on the floor; she was also thrown down concrete stairs and hit a concrete wall at the bottom of the stairs with no medical attention, which has caused brain damage. My middle daughter had gone through many tests when she was 4, for brain damage and she was place on Ritalin at age 4, and diagnosed as mentally retarded at age 9 and borderline personality disorder at age 18. She has been so hard to deal with; her behavior has been so out of control: several times I have had to call the police but they told me since she is not being abused there is nothing that they can do. I did all that I could do that I had to give up guardianship a few years ago because I could not handle it any more. She is 27 and still requires 24/7/365 care.

Since I got out of the Navy, in 1992, I have been homeless 5 times and have moved 13 times because I didn't feel comfortable where I was living. I've had at least 16 jobs since I have been out of the Navy. I have not ever worked in the field of social work, which I have my degree in.

ANONYMOUS, U.S. COAST GUARD

A Coastie had poker night at his house. Only three Coasties attended. The other Coastie was the designated driver because he is a Mormon and does not drink nor does he even play poker. Now that I think about it I am not even sure why he attended. Knowing that I didn't have to worry about driving myself home, I drank and had a good time.

The designated driver pulled into a parking lot of an office complex. It was evening on a Saturday and the parking lot was dark and empty. He told me to get out of the car. I asked him why and he said to just do it. I didn't think much about it. He told me to sit down on the ground. I thought it was weird but did it anyway. He raped me.

After he finished with me he told me to get back into his car. I was very numb and I did what he told me to. He drove me to his home. At his house he raped me again. He then told me to wash myself. He called me a dirty slut and told me that I should be ashamed at myself for having sex in public. He said that all women are sluts. He was very angry. He kept on swearing at me about how slutty and promiscuous I was and how much I should hate myself for it.

As instructed I took a shower at his house. I was numbed and scared.

He told me to get back into his car. I don't remember much after that.

Somehow I ended up at home. I woke up on my bed naked. I was still obviously very drunk. I didn't want to tell anyone because I felt very ashamed.

Everybody loves the rapist. He's the one that is always kissing everyone's ass. Not to mention he is a of higher rank than me. I wasn't going to report him.

I kept the rape to myself, not telling a soul. One night I was home and felt as if I was reliving the assault all over again. I went online and found out about RAINN. I did their online chat and they told me that they don't have listed any support from the Coast Guard in my state. They told me instead to talk to the National Guard and gave me a contact number. After talking to RAINN for a while I was able to feel more calm and it helped me.

I did not call the National Guard right away. I was very hesitant to talk to anyone. I liked RAINN because I was able to remain anonymous at the online chat but picking up the phone and talking to someone was very scary for me. Several weeks later I felt the same feeling like I was reliving the rape. I chatted with RAINN again and they told me the same thing as last time.

I looked at the National Guard website and was able to pull out the email address of the SARC that they gave me the number to. I set up an anonymous email account and emailed the SARC. She responded right away and said that she can certainly help me even though I am in the Coast Guard. She told me to call her. I waited a few weeks to call her but glad that I finally did!

First few phone calls I was hesitant to even give her my real name. She did not care. She said that she understood and was very nice to me. I was afraid that she would tell the Coast Guard what happened and that I'll lose my career! I told her about how I feel like I am being raped all over again. She says that it is very common and it is called a flashback. We probably talked six times on the phone; still I was anonymous until I gained the courage to give her my real identity and meet with her in person.

I also emailed the Coast Guard SARC but never received a response. One day I got a sudden burst of bravery and called the Coast Guard SARC in my district but since I refused to give my name I was hung up on. Picking up the phone and saying: "Hello. My name is so and so and I do not know you but I want to report a rape" is freaking hard! Why can't they understand that? Sometimes saying "Hello. I rather be anonymous for now. I was raped. What can you do for me?" is much easier. I do not know if this is a Coast Guard policy or just this specific SARC has a paranoia problem. Either way why was the National Guard able to talk to me when I did not feel comfortable sharing my name but not the Coast Guard?

The National Guard SARC said that everything that I tell her would be kept confidential and I have nothing to worry about with my command finding out. She was very nice. I opened up to her. She definitely wanted to help me. I told her about what I knew about how the Coast Guard treated rape survivors. I even told her about the Coast Guard SARC. She says that she only heard nightmares coming out of the Coast Guard and now she is seeing it firsthand. She says she agrees that the Coast Guard is not doing their part to help rape survivors but since I came to her through RAINN that she would treat me the same way she treats those in the Guard. What kind of reputation does the Coast Guard have?

She set me up with counseling. I did not like the counselor. It was nothing that the counselor did wrong except it was just not a good fit for me. The SARC right away got me an appointment with another counselor, who I felt very comfortable talking to and who I still see today. I really like how she took into account my feelings. This SARC needs to win SARC of the year. She has been great!

The SARC also recommended that I talk to the Military Rape Crisis Center because they are pretty much the experts when it comes to Coast Guard rape. I emailed them with my fake email address and they also reassured me that it is all confidential. After several weeks of them helping me without even knowing who I was, I finally disclosed my real identity. They hooked me up with a yoga program specifically for those with PTSD that I am trying my best to continue going because I know it'll be helpful. It is hard to go and be around other people. I became very isolated since the rape. I don't even want to leave my home most days.

Earlier this week we received an email from the vice-commandant for Sexual Assault Awareness Month. The rapist made a huge deal about it and said that it is horrible that women are being raped. He printed out the poster and put one on everyone's desk. It makes me want to barf. I serve with a bunch of people that start every rape-prevention discussion with: "Many women would lie about rape." I am diagnosed with Post Traumatic Stress Disorder. Every evening I drink until I black out. I can't sleep any other way. I am afraid to even leave my house. I go to work. I come home and repeat it 5 days a week. On days off I stay home. I do not know how much longer I can go through with this. Every day is a struggle. I cannot do this any longer. I give up.

S.J., U.S. AIR FORCE

It all began in March 2003. I landed in a foreign land as a technical school graduate. After departing my flight, I got settled into this new land called Okinawa. When I finally got acclimated to the shop I met my first supervisor, Staff Sergeant ★★★★★ Our first supervisor/trainee session was at CoCo's, the local curry shop. Since this was all new to me, I thought that this was how bonds were built between the ranks. Then ★★★★ began telling me about all of his heterosexual and homosexual relationships he had been having on the island. Mind you, this man was married with a child. I began to feel like this encounter was not going as it should and was feeling very uncomfortable about the topic.

After our food came he propositioned me. He said, "If you have sex with me I will give you a five out of five on your performance report. If not, I will give you a one and take away all hopes of your having any type of successful career in the military." I held off on his advances. Every day I worked with him was a day I would dread. He would ask questions such as: "If this tool were my penis, what would you do with it?" I avoided him at all costs. There was only one other female in the shop. One day we were having a drink and ★★★★'s name was mentioned and I told her what was going on. Later she informed the flight chief without my knowledge. The next thing I knew, I was being questioned in the flight chief's office and I told him everything that was going on. He changed my shift and supervisor. Then he swept the incident under the rug because it was clear that Staff Sergeant ★★★★ was the flight's golden child who received all of the awards.

I'm not quite sure whether I developed an allergy to jet fuel or if it had something to do with all the stress I was under in my shop. Either way, I could no longer do my duty as a fuel system mechanic. In October I began working for the squadron doing odds and ends jobs. In March the dorm needed an escort to take Okinawans in and out of the dorm rooms so they could work on the fire-suppression system. I began working with the contractors and one of the men began to become very friendly with me. I just ignored his behavior, not seeing him as threatening. He would point to his penis and say "piku, piku." I ignored him because I didn't know what that meant.

Then on 29 March 2004 we went to room 145 of building 600. I was reading a PlayStation magazine article about a samurai video game. He came over and asked to look at the article. I showed it to him and he took his phone out and showed me a picture of his baby daughter. Then he put his phone away and grabbed my shoulders and started to rub them. I pushed his hands away and made an "X" with my arms and told him to go back to work. Then he grabbed my breasts and began rubbing them. I made an "X" with my arms and told him no and to go back to work. Then he grabbed for my BDU (battle dress uniform) pants and unbuttoned them and began stroking my groin area with his fingers. I pushed him away and made an "X" and told him to work. Then I pulled out my phone and texted my boyfriend at the time, who then stayed with me the rest of the shift. That was on a Friday. On Monday, my boyfriend informed the dorm chief what had transpired on Friday.

I begged to speak with my first sergeant but was denied. First the dorm chief spoke with the lead contractor. He brushed it off. Then she received approval from her squadron to call the security forces and they showed up along with the Okinawan police. I identified my attacker out of a lineup and continued asking to speak with my first sergeant. Then the Okinawan police took me back to the room and had me reenact everything while they took pictures. At this point I still had not seen or spoken with my first sergeant and the Okinawan police took me to their police station. They allowed no English-speaking person to be with me at any time. My squadron commander, first sergeant, and flight chief were all too busy to come to the police station to find out what was going on. So the squadron sent a random staff sergeant whom I had never met to assist me in any way he could. Once again I had to identify my attacker from another lineup. I gave my statement and signed something that I think was what I had said to the police officers; however, I wasn't sure because it was all in kanji, the written language of Japan.

After the Okinawan police had finished their questioning, I had to go to the Military Law Enforcement Desk, which instructed me to return the next day. When I returned, I had to first give my statement to a detective, and then I had to write my statement out completely. After all that, I was finally allowed to see my first sergeant. After I began talking to the first sergeant, he pulled me into the commander's office. My commander told me I was too emotional for the situation and that he didn't want me in "his" military. He then called the mental health clinic and began asking how he could get me discharged from the military. So the process of being separated from the Service began while I was dealing with the sexual assault. After that I met with the military prosecutor and again told the details of my traumatic event. Finally I made it to the Okinawan prosecutor. He told me the man who had sexually assaulted me would not be tried.

I was told by this prosecutor that it was my attacker's first time and that because his wife had just had a baby, what he had done to me was okay. At this juncture, the people above me tried discharging me from the military on two separate occasions and they failed each time. After three years in Japan, I was sent to McChord AFB in Lakewood, WA. I was working with a therapist on getting over my trauma overseas. And then, while at home one day, I was raped. I was the head coach of the squadron soccer team and one of the players was a master sergeant in my flight. There had been a couple of complaints about his behavior to Military Equal Opportunity, information I wish I had known beforehand. On the last Friday of April we played a hard game and lost, not surprising since we didn't win any games that season. I went home as usual, cleaned up, and sprawled out on my futon to watch a movie.

I received a couple of phone calls from a Master Sergeant **** asking me to go out to a bar with him. I told him no and that I was going to sleep. Around 10:00 p.m. I received a knock on the door. I looked out the peephole, saw that it was Master Sergeant ****, and, thinking something important was going on, I opened the door. From that point on my life was in fast forward to pause to slow motion to the end. When I opened the door I could smell the booze on his breath. He grabbed my arm and took me to my bedroom. He threw me on my bed and tore off my clothes. He held a knife to my throat. I asked him what he was doing. He didn't answer.

Then I froze. Within a split second, I had flashbacks of every trauma I had ever experienced. Then he was on top of me with his pants down and he began the act of raping me. He first began by inserting his penis into my vagina. It seemed like he was rocking back and forth forever. Then he told me to tell him that I wanted him to cum inside me. Wanting things to end, I said it. Then he came. Then he flipped me over and began to sodomize me. I just remember the pain and then him telling me to say the same phrase to him again. So I complied again. He pulled his black boxers and black Levis up. He then hit me a couple of times and told me no one must know of our relationship. So I kept quiet.

About the end of May I had been drinking and when someone mentioned Master Sergeant ***, I began to cry and told them I had been raped by him. Little did I know that by revealing this information, I would eventually be victimized again by deceit and falsehoods. In late July my commander promised to hold my hand during an entire Office of Special Investigations inquiry. I believed her, but unfortunately that turned out to be a blatant lie. When I finally gathered up enough courage to talk to the investigators, I let them know all that had happened. They did their investigation and then they called Master Sergeant **** in for questioning. He claimed that on the night in question, the team was going to a bar to hang out. He said he went to my place to pick me up to go with, but that I had told him I didn't want to go and that we sat and had a drink. Once the commander heard his story she backed away from me and said she couldn't choose sides. She then told me that his wife had just had a baby and that this was his first offense. She then assigned Master Sergeant **** to a workstation 100 yards away from mine, which meant that I would have to see him each and every day when I left or came to work. Some days he would approach me and I would have anxiety attacks. Other times I was forced to be in the same room with him. That year I was hospitalized in the psychiatric unit seven separate times. The commander grew angry and told me that I needed to have bearing and to start behaving like a good airman.

After being hospitalized a few times I lost all faith in the military and its elite brotherhood through thick and thin and requested a medical discharge. I missed out on making rank—something I had been looking forward to—but I thought I would be able to stop reliving the trauma with the military no longer there. That did not work. Sometimes I get down on myself, thinking, *I didn't go to war so why do I get to be a veteran?* I did what only 1 percent of the general population does. I signed that dotted line and said I would march into battle for my country if called upon. I just wasn't called upon. Because of the traumatic experiences I had on the homefront, I had to take care of that first before they would send me to any more traumatic places, which is why I still am a veteran. I am proud to be a veteran. I think all veterans should be proud. I've been in inpatient psychiatric units on approximately 10 separate occasions. When you are in the inpatient unit, you are stripped of everything, given pajamas to wear all day, and are medicated. When you're in the unit you cannot leave for any reason other than a discharge. There is a possibility that you can be put into four-point restraints. Once you become stable enough to return to real life, they then release you. But what is real life when you live with post-traumatic stress disorder?

EXAMPLES OF VA SCREENING TO IDENTIFY SEXUAL TRAUMA

Grace

Grace is a 33-year-old married mother of two and a Gulf War veteran, in for her annual checkup. She has no complaints. With the door closed, the nurse reviews the clinical reminders and Grace's self-administered questionnaire. The nurse, making eye contact, slowly and calmly continues:

Nurse: "One of the questions we now ask all veterans pertains to their military experiences, primarily negative experiences like unwanted sexual attention or forced sexual experiences. During your military experience, did anyone ever force you to have unwanted sexual contact OR did anyone ever repeatedly do any of the following: ask for sexual favors, pressure you for sex, corner you, make sexist jokes, or demean you because you were female?"

Grace: "Why are you asking about things like that?"

Nurse: "The VA is very concerned about those types of experiences and the effect they can have on people's health. We also have specialized services to help those veterans who want help addressing any health issues related to such experiences."

Grace stares at the wall and informs the nurse about an episode of date rape during her military experience, which she did not report and for which she did not seek medical attention. However, she did discuss the situation with her close friend. She reports having difficulty sleeping for a month after the date rape.

Grace: "I was assaulted once but I was in the wrong place at the wrong time with the wrong guy. I was drunk, off-base at the time, and on a date with this guy who ended up being a jerk."

Making eye contact, the nurse empathically states, "I'm sorry that happened. Unfortunately, experiences like that happen too frequently, and what you experienced would be called, 'military sexual trauma.' We have special services available for those who want them."

The nurse tells Grace about the type of services provided: "Oh, things like counseling, talk therapy, psychiatry, medical care for related medical issues."

Grace: "Hmmm, interesting. Well, I had problems right after it happened, but after about 6 months and talking my best friend's ear off (smiles), I'm certainly OK now. I'm happy, have a great family, love my job, and don't have any real health issues."

Nurse: "That's great." The nurse smiles back. "I will document that you have experienced what we call military sexual trauma, but the information will be kept confidential. You shouldn't be asked again about such experiences. If, at any time in the future, you wish to talk about your experience, please let us know so we can get the right staff involved."

The nurse continues on, "Let's complete the rest of these questions, okay?"

After completing the questions, the nurse enters all the information into the Computerized Patient Record System (CPRS) and gives Grace a locally developed brochure about MST.

During the physical exam with her usual primary care provider, Grace spontaneously relays the MST experience to her female primary care provider.

Grace: "You know, it's so nice that VA has special services for women who've been raped in the military."

The provider concurs: "Yes, we've developed some unique services that any veteran can access."

The provider pauses, makes direct eye contact with Grace, and asks, "If you want to talk with anyone about your experience, just let me know, okay?"

Grace nods.

Provider: "You know it's common that women have more than one such experience, or end up in unhappy relationships. Has that happened with you?"

Grace: "No, I just had the one experience. And my husband is a dear."

Provider: "So, you feel happy and safe with your husband?"

Grace: "Yes."

One week later, Grace calls the clinic and talks with the nurse.

Grace: "You know, I went home and read that brochure you gave me. It mentions something about benefits. Can you tell me more about that?"

The nurse briefly relays the VBA claims process and suggests contacting the veterans service officer at the local VA Regional Office or facility MST coordinator for more information. She sends additional information to Grace. Grace never files a claim, but she shares this "new" information with some women she knows who served in the military.

Kevin

Kevin is a 53-year-old, unemployed, divorced, Vietnam-era veteran who uses tobacco and drinks alcohol excessively. He has been medically hospitalized at least once for severe alcohol-related withdrawal symptoms. His medical problems include hypertension, chronic obstructive pulmonary disease, and chronic hepatitis C. Some progress notes describe Kevin as "having difficulty with interpersonal relationships." Kevin's VA medical record documents his medical problems and the general overview of his childhood and Military Services. No mention of violence or abuse exists in his medical record.

Presenting Problem:

Kevin presents with abdominal pain. His provider is out sick. In the past, he has refused to be seen by a medical resident in training. He doesn't want to wait to be evaluated and reluctantly agrees to be seen by a female resident.

The nurse ushers Kevin into an exam room and quickly takes his vitals and asks him the reason for his visit ("I need to talk with someone about this pain").

The nurse meets the covering resident in the hallway and mentions that Kevin is ready to be seen, that his vitals are "OK," and that he wants to talk about abdominal pain.

The resident enters the room shortly thereafter, introduces herself politely and shakes his hand, and then sits down near Kevin.

> *Resident:* "Give me a minute here, while I bring up your record. Then we can get down to business."

She signs onto CPRS, bringing up Kevin's record. Quickly noting Kevin's problem list, she scans the last progress note from the attending and the clinical reminders that are due. Colorectal cancer screening and MST are the only visible clinical reminders. She calmly turns to Kevin and begins asking about his abdominal pain, which has been occurring intermittently since he was discharged from the military, but is progressing in severity. She completes a review of systems targeting abdominal pain, with negative results, but also has Kevin agree to complete the colorectal cancer screening. She then asks about his use of alcohol.

> *Kevin:* "Nah, I've been trying to avoid that stuff. It's caused too many problems in my life. You know, it's really hard to quit drinking. I keep relapsing, but this time, I think I've got it. I've finally started attending AA about a month ago and haven't had a drink since."
>
> *Resident:* "That's great, when did you start drinking?"
>
> *Kevin (guardedly):* "When I was stationed in Vietnam."
>
> *Resident:* "May I ask why you started using alcohol?"
>
> Kevin gruffly states, "Aren't you getting a little personal here?"
>
> The resident meets Kevin's agitated eyes calmly and warmly. "I'm here to help figure out what your pain is from so we can try to make it better. Alcohol may be a factor so I'm asking."

Kevin nods, his face relaxing somewhat.

The resident pauses and continues: "People start using alcohol for many reasons, including peer pressure and to deal with stressful situations. Might that be true for you?"

Kevin sighs, staring at the ceiling: "Maybe."

The resident recognizes the opportunity and goes on. "Some people have had stressful, negative experiences in the military, including unwanted sexual experiences and unwanted sexual attention. Did anything like that happen to you?"

Kevin closes his eyes tightly, but it doesn't stop the tears that slowly trickle down his face.

Resident: "Do you want to talk about it?" The resident asks quietly, avoiding the temptation to reach out and touch Kevin's hand lying on the desk.

A prolonged silence commences.

Kevin: "No, I don't think I want to talk."

Resident: "Well, if you do, you don't have to go into detail. That might be too hard."

Kevin then slowly says, his voice breaking, "You know, I've never had anyone ask me about that, not even my usual doc. And I've never told anyone about what happened."

Resident: "Are you telling me that you had such an experience?"

Kevin nods purposefully, tears still flowing, but looking directly at the resident.

She continues in an empathic tone. "I'm sorry that happened. You know those kind of experiences happened to a lot of men and women in the military. And we have special services for those people who want them."

Another pause follows.

Kevin: "I always thought that I could use the alcohol to chase away the nightmares, the anxiety, the feeling that it would happen again. . . ."

Resident: "Have you been having those reactions recently?"

Kevin: "Yes"—wiping away the tears—"and I'm scared that I'll start drinking again, but I don't know how to get rid of the nightmares, and the pain in my gut. Every time I begin thinking about it, the pain comes and I can barely stand it. I mean the pain is starting now."

Resident: "I think we can help you."

The resident briefly mentions that physical pain is sometimes related to other kinds of pain. She tells him that treatment is available, that medications might also help reduce his anxiety and nightmares. She reassures him that confidentiality will be maintained as much as possible.

Kevin relaxes some more, but appears skeptical.

Resident: "If you want, we can use some initial medicine to control the anxiety and hopefully the nightmares. That might also help with the abdominal pain; if not, we can try something else. It might be very helpful if you talked with a specialist about what happened. I've seen many veterans benefit from seeing a specialist. If you want, I can get a specialist involved."

Kevin: "Let me think about it."

Resident: "No problem. Here's a brochure that explains more about what we call military sexual trauma and the services we offer."

Kevin: "I know. I've read the brochures out in the waiting room about a dozen times and was wondering if anyone would ever ask me, and how I'd react. Now I know. You think it'll help?"

The resident nods.

Kevin: "Well, let's give that medicine you mentioned a try." He pauses, and then continues, "Yeah, let's get that specialist involved. Is it going to be a guy? Cause if it's a guy, I'm not interested!"

The resident reassures him that a female counselor can be requested. The referral is made. The veteran is given some trazodone to try at bedtime. An appointment is made for follow-up in one month, with the resident, at Kevin's request.

Kevin keeps the appointment with the MST counselor, a female. He also returns for his follow-up with the resident. After six months, Kevin quietly transfers his medical care totally to the resident. Kevin continues to abstain from alcohol, but does agree to have psychiatry involved in his care, also, where an SSRI is added to his trazodone. He is diagnosed with chronic, complex PTSD. His abdominal pain lessens, and then disappears in about six months. The nightmares and anxiety also lessen.

Eighteen months later, Kevin's abdominal pain returns and worsens. The resident, now an attending, sees him in her Continuing Care Clinic. She completes a review of systems with negative results. He remains abstinent from alcohol and hasn't used illicit drugs.

Provider: "What else has been going on in your life?"

Kevin: "Well, nothing's changed, if that's what you're asking. I still see the counselor, the psychiatrist, and attend AA. My kids and grandchildren see me more often." He pauses, and then states, "Now that I think of it, I have filed a VA disability claim. But that shouldn't make a difference."

Provider: "Have you told your counselor or your psychiatrist that you've filed a VA claim?"

Kevin: "No, it's none of their business. They might think that I'm just trying to get money."

The provider then explains that physical symptoms can worsen when a disability claim is filed, but that improvement is usually seen when the claim is completed. She stresses the importance of involving his other healthcare providers in his care during this time. Kevin agrees to talk with his other providers about filing a disability claim.

ANATOMY OF AN ASSAULT

The following is a case study used by the Center for the Army Profession and Ethic (CAPE), http://cape.army.mil, to enable small-group discussion about how the crime of sexual assault and a culture that enables sexual harassment contradict all essential characteristics of the Army profession.

PFC Schuette was the victim of sexual assault and sexual harassment during her basic training. The perpetrator was her drill sergeant, who was found guilty of multiple crimes and sentenced to five years in prison. She chose to continue serving and is currently stationed at Fort Bragg, North Carolina. She shares her experience because she wants to ensure other soldiers don't experience the same physical trauma and mental anguish. She wants to inspire everyone to report any incident involving sexual assault and harassment. These are her own words.

First Signs of Unprofessional Behavior

When we got back from Christmas, that was when everything kind of started to lay into place that was not right. And a particular drill sergeant, who called me out sometimes during stuff, had a specific nickname for me, which was "TJ." He called me out a lot more to sing in front of the formations. Um, he would pick on me a lot more. He picked on a few other privates a lot more. I noticed him kind of singling out people more. He would start off little with something and see if you would say anything or do anything, see if you would tell other privates. It all kind of worked its way into what it became. But he was very, very sly. He was mastermind at it.

Red Flags

I had one occasion where a battle buddy and I, we were running down the stairs, and a particular drill sergeant . . . he yelled down the stairwell and he was like, "Hey Privates," and . . . the battle buddy in front of me was down a step where she couldn't see him. And as he was talking to her, um, he was making kissing and winking faces at me and so that would have been my first red flag. We ran back down to formation and I was like, "Battle Buddy, this just happened," and she was like, "I didn't see it," so we really couldn't report it and we really couldn't say anything about it. It was just one thing that had happened.

I was out on the firing range and the same drill sergeant came around and as he cleared my weapon, he was asking me if, if I would let him have sex with me or if there was anybody in the barracks that he could. Um, and I was, I was so shocked. I was like, "No, drill sergeant. You know, I don't know if anybody in the bay would, would wanna do that." I said, you know, "No." When I got back I went to that same battle buddy. She and I talked about it and she was like, "Wow, I can't believe he said that." And there was nobody around though because the firing range was set up differently. And, um, so there was no, again no witnesses for anything. But that would have been my second red flag.

The Assault

The next day was then when the actual assault happened. We were pulling everything out and were doing an inventory for everything for a change of command. So, as we're pulling things out, he had yelled from his office . . . "Hey TJ." So I came into his office and that was when the actual assault happened. He had kind of cornered me and he, he knew what he could do where other privates wouldn't see from the bay. After the assault had happened I ran out and I was, oh I was looking for a battle buddy to go over to the other bay cuz I knew I needed to tell somebody. And I was crying hysterically and everybody was so worried about what they were doing they didn't, they didn't really stop and pay attention to me. Like what had just happened or asked me what was going on. I was absolutely just mortified. I was terrified. I had no idea what to do.

And I went and I talked to this battle buddy and she was like, "You've got to tell somebody." But we didn't know who.

Seeking Help

We were very stuck on who, who we trusted, who we thought would help us. We are on basic training. We are new to the rank system. We don't understand everything; we don't understand the army. And so we took a little bit of a, a little bit of an opportunity to kinda, kinda brainstorm and kind of think about what was going on. Even though I was still absolutely hysterical and I was, oh, I was so lost. We had then had the opportunity to go the PX during that day.

And while we were there it, it was just eating me alive. And I just, I couldn't, couldn't keep it together and I had just started bawling. And then everybody, it became more apparent that there was really something wrong, cuz I am a very outgoing person and there was definitely something wrong.

Misplaced Loyalty

More privates kind of got involved. Um, one particular one was a male private and he heard my story and he was very good friends with the drill sergeant who had done this. So as soon as we got back from the PX he ran up there and told that drill sergeant that I was gonna tell on him. And that was when stuff got kind of crazy. Um, as soon as he found out, he started throwing stuff in his office. Oh, he was swearing up and down the ____. He said, "You bring her in here." And I was like, "I am not going over there. That is not gonna happen. He can come over here and yell at me with all these privates in this room. He can come over here. I'm not going over there where there's nobody over there." Um, so those privates went over there and told him that and he came back and said that he was gonna come drag me by my hair if I didn't go over there. I said I would like to request to talk to a different drill sergeant. And that was when another drill sergeant came up and he pulled me into that office and I had told him everything that had happened. And he pretty much asked me if I wanted to open up that can of worms. He said that is my battle buddy's career that you're about to mess with. Um, he asked me if I was dreaming. He asked me if I was lying. Um, he brought in another drill sergeant who was one of my other ones and that drill sergeant was like, "You know we should really report this." So they did. They called the first sergeant.

Trust between Soldiers and Leaders

It was on a weekend. She was not very happy about coming in on the weekend. So when she came in, she was pretty hot. She came in there, she questioned all three of us, and then she had all three of us write statements. They read through them and they made the determination that this drill sergeant wasn't smart enough to do this. That he didn't have any reason why he would do this. He has a family. He has a wife. So, they went with the fact that they were just gonna keep it at company level and kind of sweep it underneath the rug. And they didn't, didn't believe me at all. They, the next day they tried to tell me that I was getting chaptered out for having a lack of integrity. Um, they moved me to a different platoon and that platoon absolutely, none of the drill sergeants liked me at all. They all, they all harassed me; they all hazed me. They all had their own opinions of what, what happened. They all thought he was a stellar drill sergeant.

Earning Trust

During the next day we were doing combatives and this sergeant major walked by and I was like this is it cuz I, there's nothing else, nobody's gonna do for me. So I went and I talked to sergeant-major and he, he, he finally put his foot down. And he brought all the females up to that bay. He said, "I need to know what's going on. I need to know if this drill sergeant is doing anything to anybody. Because right now I have a private with an allegation and nobody's gonna believe her unless there's more." And finally people broke. Finally we had hands all over the room. We had comments that he had said that were inappropriate. You know, behavior that he shouldn't have done and there were also some rape cases.

Lost Faith in the Profession

When I approached the sergeant-major I really had no idea if he would be able to help me or if he had any idea of what was going on. I pretty much was going off of a, going off of a blank sheet, just hoping that somebody would listen. By then I had lost faith in every single person that was wearing this uniform.

Competence over Character

During the time where the investigation was going on, a lot of the males really, really stuck with this drill sergeant. They really thought he was great. Um, he really was a good drill sergeant. He taught us the basics of survival instead of sitting there doing the silly stuff, pushups and stuff. He was very good, ah, with tactical stuff, with life-saving things. Um, so a lot of people, they did stick behind him during this. But, honestly by then I was, if you didn't like me, don't talk to me.

Um, many times people, people look at just the outside, you know, competence that somebody has, and the outside character and the outside way that a person presents themself; from the outside this drill sergeant was stellar. He was fast-tracking on his way to first sergeant. He really was. Um, a lot of times people miss, they miss the, the singling-out stuff, and they miss him pulling females to the side. Cuz if you're a male, you don't, you don't particularly pay attention to that. Us females, we kinda try to stick together as a team once somebody kind of said something. "Hey this guy's kinda creepy." We all kinda gathered on that bandwagon to kinda look out for each other. But if you're, if you're a male and you're not noticing it, you're kind of lost and you really just kind of think of him as a stellar soldier.

Trust between Soldiers

Um, there were many things I could have done. Um, we thought about, thought about talking to the chaplain. We thought about talking to a drill sergeant. We thought about not saying a word. I confided in more than one person, which definitely helped me get a little bit more of a view. A lot of the motivation to keep going would be from my battle buddies. Um, they offered to move me to a different company to get me away from everybody in that unit, all the drill sergeants and everything, but I opted to stay there because really during those, those three or four days where I was just absolutely hounded on, those females really, we really got a tight connection. And, um, that's what the army's all about.

The Effect on Trust

As a private, um, and being demeaned by so many, so many higher-ranking NCOs, especially male and female, kind of definitely has affected me in many ways. Um, just even being here, I, I definitely act differently toward male NCOs. Like it's, it's, it just happens. I have no control over it. If they approach me in a wrong way or if they say, "Hey, you know, this needs to be better," I take that personally instead of as a soldier. When it comes to trusting chain of command, you definitely say I have a little bit of issues with that as well. I am like the first person to run up to somebody higher and skip that middle person because to me that was, that was the only way anybody heard me was to skip all the way up to a sergeant-major. So that was, that was kind of the way that now is triggered in my brain that stuff will get done when really it should be, you know, keep it at the lowest level.

Personal Courage

I was not the only person, um, that this drill sergeant had victimized. There were many and there was many in that same unit with me in that same bay.

Once I had came forward, they saw what I had went through, all the hazing, all the harassment, and they were terrified. Those, those other females had made a pact not to say anything. They weren't gonna say anything till the day they died. They were gonna let me sink.

I have asked them, you know, where did you come from and how did, how did your situation happen, and why didn't you say anything? And they just, they all had said that they were not strong enough. They didn't feel like they could trust anybody there and they didn't want to put themselves out there and have people look at 'em funny. You know, they, they were scared. They were just like any other person would be. I was scared. Um, but when it came down to it, they really just wanted to know that somebody was gonna do something. Of course you're not gonna say anything if, if somebody higher up is telling you that they're gonna rip your rank off and kick you out. So early in the game, that may be all you have. You came into the army with the army. So a lot of times, people, I know from their situation they were very scared that they would lose their career.

Trust between Soldiers and the Army

While I did have the option to get out of the army, um, I choose not to. I decided that, you know, my, my father was prior military. My grandfather was prior military. My other grandfather was. It's not, it's not the Army. It is the person that did this and the people that followed him, that had bad judgment. The military doesn't tell you to take away your morals and your standards. Sometimes people just forget when they put on that rank that maybe, maybe this isn't right, or maybe they're using their rank for their own advantages.

Be Passionate and Approachable

The training that we had, um, was very interesting. In the first couple weeks we get there, they compile every little single little thing that they need to throw at you in a PowerPoint, death by PowerPoint. We had so many slideshows to go through: EO, SHARP, how to do this, how to do that. Um, when it came down to it, I honestly can't remember one thing particular that came from any of the videos at all because we were so tired, and we were so beat down, and none of those videos helped me at all.

The SHARP program definitely could have been enhanced if they had maybe a live speaker talk about it, or if they just had somebody that was passionate about it. I think that's where a lot of times it gets kind of get thrown under the rug. We just make people the SHARP, but they're not passionate about it. They have no desire to, to really get with victims and see how, how they operate because you can't really fix something that's a problem if you don't understand where that person may be coming from. A lot of the times I've run into a few that just, they're not approachable. As a victim, you need to be approachable. If I can't approach you with my deepest, darkest secrets, you are nothing. You, you are of no help. All the training you have is nothing if I don't come forward.

Moral Courage

For other soldiers out there, for this, you know, any, any sort of harassment or assault or rape, bring it to somebody's attention. It doesn't matter who, just somebody because it will eat you alive. It will stay in you and nobody can walk around with that for the rest of their lives and not be miserable. Like you have to tell somebody about it. Um, that way something can be done if there are repercussions from it. There are proper, ah, steps that say that that is not allowed. Um, I just want people to know that there are others out there like myself. There are; you're not alone.

II

6

SOLUTIONS

In January 2012, the Department revised and reissued DoDD 6495.01, which included a requirement that the Military Services align their prevention strategies with the DoD Sexual Assault Prevention Strategy. The central tenet of this strategy is the Spectrum of Prevention, which describes six levels of influence and intervention, ranging from individuals to organization-wide policy.

THE SPECTRUM OF PREVENTION

By addressing sexual assault prevention at each of the six levels in military society, the Department seeks to promote a culture where all members of the DoD community understand their role in prevention and act to reduce the occurrence of sexual assault in the military.

In order to improve military commanders' understanding of the prevention culture and climate within their units, DoD SAPRO and Defense Manpower Data Center (DMDC) worked with the Defense Equal Opportunity Management Institute (DEOMI) to develop six SAPR-focused questions for inclusion in the Defense Equal Opportunity Climate Survey (DEOCS) and Air Force Unit Climate Assessment surveys. These surveys provide commanders with a real-time assessment of their command climate related to discriminatory attitudes and behaviors.

Included among the new SAPR questions are two questions that specifically address the propensity for unit members to intervene in situations at risk for sexual assault. The two questions allow a commander to assess how well unit members understand prevention concepts and whether or not members feel empowered to act in a given situation. One question is

Table 6.1.

Influencing Policy and Legislation
Changing Organizational Practices
Fostering Coalitions and Networks
Educating Providers
Promoting Community Education
Strengthening Individual Knowledge and Skills

situation-based and asks respondents to indicate *which action* they would take if in a given situation.

Q. Suppose you see a Service member put something in a person's drink. You're unsure what it was and question if your eyes were playing tricks on you. What are you most likely to do in this kind of situation?

Confront the Service member.
Tell the person what you saw the Service member do.
Watch the situation to see if it escalates.
Leave to avoid any kind of trouble.
Nothing.

The second question presents a scenario to respondents and asks at *which point they would most likely intervene* if they witnessed the escalating situation.

Q. Imagine you go temporary duty (TDY) for some training. The first night you go to a restaurant/bar with a large group of colleagues, whom you just met. At what point would you intervene in the following escalating situation?

A senior leader at the training buys your colleague a drink and he/she is told a drink may never be refused, as doing so would go against tradition.

The senior leader buys your colleague a second and third drink despite his/her repeated objections.

Your colleague appears intoxicated and disoriented, and continues to be the senior leader's main focus of attention.

The senior leader repeatedly hugs your colleague, rubs his/her shoulders, and offers to walk him/her back to quarters.

You see the senior leader quietly taking your intoxicated colleague out of the place.

As they leave, your colleague tries to push away the senior leader and says, "No."

In this scenario, I would not intervene at any point.

INCREASING THE CLIMATE OF VICTIM CONFIDENCE

A top priority is to increase the number of victims making a report of sexual assault. The Department seeks to increase the reporting rate by improving the confidence that service members have in the military justice process, ensuring they receive the support they desire during this process, enhancing the education they receive about reporting options, and reducing stigma and other barriers that deter reporting.

In FY12, there were 3,374 reports of sexual assault involving service members. This represents a 6 percent increase over the 3,192 reports of sexual assault received in FY11. The 3,374 reports received in FY12 involved 2,949 service member victims.

Due to the underreporting of this crime in both military and civilian society, reports to authorities do not necessarily equate to the actual prevalence (occurrence) of sexual assault. In fact, the Department estimates that about 11 percent of the sexual assaults that occur each year are reported to a DoD authority. This is roughly the same pattern of underreporting seen in other segments of civilian society. Underreporting of sexual assault interferes with the Department's efforts to provide victims with needed care and its ability to hold offenders appropriately accountable.

Concerns about loss of privacy and negative scrutiny by others often act as barriers that keep civilian and military victims from reporting. According to the *2012 WGRA*, of the active-duty women who indicated experiencing unwanted sexual contact (USC) and did not report it to a military authority, the top three reasons for not reporting were as follows:

70 percent did not want anyone to know;
66 percent felt uncomfortable making a report; and
51 percent did not think the report would be kept confidential.

Due to the relatively small numbers of active-duty men who indicated experiencing USC and did not report it to a military authority, there was considerable variance in the responses and most responses were not reportable. However, the three reasons for which data was reportable were:

22 percent believed they or others would be punished for other infractions or violations, such as underage drinking;
17 percent thought they would not be believed; and
16 percent thought their performance evaluation or chance for promotion would suffer.

In 2012, the President signed an executive order establishing Military Rule of Evidence (MRE) 514, "Victim–Victim Advocate Privilege," which protects communications between victims and their SARC or SAPR VA. While there are certain exceptions, the privilege allows the victim to refuse to disclose, and prevent any other person from disclosing, confidential communications between the victim and a SAPR VA, when the communication was made for the purpose of obtaining advice or assistance. The enactment of this rule was the culmination of significant efforts by the Department to address victims' privacy concerns and promote confidence in the reporting process.

DoD SAPRO continued its efforts with other DoD entities to increase education and awareness of the Department's reporting options. DoD SAPRO collaborated with the Office of the DoD Inspector General (IG) on a prospective, voluntary, anonymous victim experience survey by supporting the development of the research instrument and methodology. The experiences of current victims will serve to inform improvements in the handling of future cases and identify additional means by which to encourage additional victim reporting.

In 2012, the Military Services and the National Guard Bureau employed a variety of means to help military personnel understand the reporting options available to sexual assault victims.

The Army made reporting a key topic in all Army training, including mandatory annual unit training, and pre- and post-deployment training. Additionally, reporting was included in SHARP training at all Army installation newcomer orientations. Local commands, leaders, and soldiers throughout the Army also spread awareness of reporting options by disseminating outreach materials on installation grounds, websites, newspapers, and public service announcements (PSA).

The Navy embarked on a heavy marketing campaign via brochures, posters, websites, and PSAs to publicize the SAPR program, including information about Restricted and Unrestricted Reporting and the DoD Safe Helpline. Navy installation websites prominently featured information describing crisis response services and reporting options.

The Marine Corps included reporting information in all SAPR training initiatives, briefs, and promotional materials. Marine Corps installation websites, newspaper articles, and 24/7 helplines also provided information on reporting options.

The Air Force leveraged its annual SAPR Leader Summit as an opportunity to reemphasize the difference between Restricted and Unrestricted Reporting and discuss the advantages and disadvantages of each option.

Examples of local efforts include the Pacific Air Forces' use of the local Commander's Access Channel and dorm safety bulletin boards to publicize SARC contact information and reporting options.

The Chief of the National Guard Bureau and Directors and senior enlisted leaders of the Army and Air National Guard released PSAs publicizing the availability of the DoD Safe Helpline as a 24/7 crisis support service across the world. Additionally, each state National Guard SAPR program provided resources to Soldiers and Airmen through PSAs, billboards, and Sexual Assault Awareness Month (SAAM) events.

Victim Confidence in the Military Justice Process

The Pentagon's own Sexual Assault Prevention and Response 2012 report showed that 62 percent of active-duty women respondents subjected to unwanted sexual contact had perceived some form of social, administrative, or professional retaliation. Another 66 percent of those victims said they felt uncomfortable making a report, and half believed nothing would be done.

"This is not a new problem, but the military for two decades has failed to solve it," said Glen Caplin, spokesman for Senator Kirsten Gillibrand (D-New York), who advocated new legislation to tackle the problem.

Taryn Meeks, executive director of Protect Our Defenders, an advocacy group for military sexual assault victims, said the military justice system needs fundamental reform, and congressional bills to deal more effectively with sexual assault within the ranks do not go far enough. Among several areas in need of reform, she said, are taking the decision to prosecute a case outside the chain of command and putting it in the hands of independent and trained JAG lawyers, and the elimination of the "good soldier" as a character defense for a convicted perpetrator.

Military juries, frequently composed of senior leaders in uniform, have often handed out "offensively light" sentences to convicted offenders, she said. In some cases, the sentences may be 60 to 90 days in confinement and the perpetrator returns to the same unit he left and where the offense occurred, she said. "What message that sends is you may be a rapist, but you're still good enough for our military," she said. "Victims have been blamed for putting themselves in a position to let assault happen," she said in an investigative article in the *Dayton Daily News* on July 7, 2013.

The military should follow the model of civilian federal courts of a judge handling sentencing and prosecutors making the determination to prosecute without the influence or veto power of unit commanders, she said.

Improving Confidence

Victims' confidence in the military justice process is believed to influence their decision to report a sexual assault and ultimately participate in military justice actions. For example, of the active-duty women who indicated on the *2012 WGRA* that they experienced USC and did not report it, 50 percent believed that nothing would be done with their report, and 43 percent heard about negative experiences other victims who reported their situation went through.

The Department's reissuance of a revised DoDD 6495.01 aimed to encourage reporting by protecting victims of sexual assault from coercion, retaliation, and reprisal in accordance with DoDD 7050.06, "Military Whistleblower Protection." In addition, it expanded the categories of persons who are eligible for Restricted Reporting to include military dependents 18 years of age and older, thus enhancing available services for an important part of the DoD community.

In an April 2012 memorandum, the secretary of defense directed that, effective June 28, 2012, in certain sexual assault cases, the initial disposition authority under the UCMJ be elevated to commanders who possess at least special court-martial convening authority and who are in the O-6 grade (i.e., colonel or Navy captain) or higher. A primary focus of this action is to put sexual assault cases under the consideration of seasoned, senior commanders who are advised by legal counsel.

In FY12, the Military Services and the National Guard Bureau successfully implemented the secretary of defense directive to elevate disposition authority. The Army enhanced implementation through annual training for soldiers, professional military education for leaders, and training for judge advocates (JA) and commanders. Finalized guidance will be included in an upcoming revision to AR 600-20, Army Command Policy.

The Navy Office of the Judge Advocate General (JAG) enhanced implementation by providing training that ensured familiarity with changes to UCMJ Article 120 and the directive's impact on the handling of sexual assault allegations.

The Marine Corps implemented and expanded the directive to also include aggravated sexual contact, abusive sexual contact, rape of a child, sexual assault of a child, sexual abuse of a child, and any attempts to commit those offenses, and for all other alleged offenses arising from or relating to the same incident.

In the National Guard, the adjutant general (O-8) holds initial disposition authority for disciplinary decisions when the matter falls outside the jurisdiction of the Army Criminal Investigative Division (CID) and the Air Force Office of Special Investigations (AFOSI), and when civilian law enforcement declines to investigate.

The Military Services and the National Guard Bureau also worked to increase victim confidence in the military justice process by developing and maintaining resources to better investigate and address allegations of sexual assault.

The Army maintained 21 special victim investigators and 19 special victim prosecutors at major Army installations who focused almost exclusively on sexual assault cases. In addition, staff JAs were required to appoint Victim-Witness Liaison personnel to advise victims of their crime victim rights, help them seek assistance, and prepare them for the military justice process.

The Naval Criminal Investigative Service (NCIS) initiated the NCIS Text & Web Tip Line, an anonymous tip-collection system that provides service members direct and real-time feedback. This service gives service members a discreet, secure, and anonymous reporting option to express concerns while minimizing fear of retaliation.

The Marine Corps published Bulletin 5813, *Detailing of Trial Counsel, Defense Counsel, and Article 32, UCMJ, Investigating Officers*, ensuring that JAs performing such functions possess the appropriate expertise to perform their duties. Additionally, NCIS conducted 389 sexual assault awareness briefings to more than 48,000 service members and civilians as part of the NCIS Crime Reduction Campaign. Ninety-five NCIS employees, special agents, investigators, and support personnel also received advanced sexual assault investigation training, which included victim interviewing and interaction techniques.

The Air Force Office of Special Investigations developed an eight-day advanced Sex Crimes Investigations Training Program (SCITP) and authored a new policy to improve agents' ability to investigate these types of crimes. SCITP attendees were taught the Cognitive Interview technique, which was designed to enhance victim and witness recall of crime details.

National Guard Bureau Instruction 0400.01 established a trained sexual assault investigator in each state and created the Judge Advocate Office of Complex Investigations, which provides an investigator upon request of the state Adjutants General. Investigators attended the Army's Sexual Assault Investigators' Course to learn how to conduct sensitive and thorough investigations of sexual assault. These investigators will document the facts in sexual assault reports when the offender is not investigated by a civilian authority and also falls outside military legal authority.

The DoD community continues to face several reporting process challenges. In deployed environments, sexual assault response procedures must be continually revised as forces redeploy within or depart the area. In addition, communication difficulties within combat zones or among geographically dispersed units have the potential to slow response to a victim in need of support.

While the Military Services and joint bases have created guidance to address sexual assault reporting and victim support at joint bases, the Department has initiated an assessment of SAPR services in joint base environments in FY13.

The Military Services have also identified challenges with maintaining confidentiality of some Restricted Reports due to the occasional improper disclosure to command by first responders. The Military Services will continue educational and training efforts to ensure service members and first responders have a clear understanding of reporting options and the exceptions to Restricted Reporting. The Military Services also identified several challenges to tracking victim services, particularly in instances when victims redeploy, move between installations or components, transition from title 10 to title 32 status, or when cases are investigated by local civilian law enforcement. The Military Services are striving to resolve these issues by enhancing coordination prior to deployment; developing relationships with off-post agencies through the implementation of written agreements; and facilitating cross-training with local agencies, including rape crisis centers, hospitals, and law enforcement. DSAID will also improve continuity of care by facilitating the transfer of cases and standardizing data collection.

7

MILITARY DISCIPLINE AND CONDUCT

POLICIES

DoDD 6495.01, January 23, 2012

SUBJECT: Sexual Assault Prevention and Response (SAPR) Program

1. PURPOSE. This Directive reissues DoD Directive (DoDD) 6495.01 (Reference (a)), pursuant to section 113 of title 10, United States Code (U.S.C.) (Reference (b)), to implement DoD policy and assign responsibilities for the SAPR Program on prevention, response, and oversight to sexual assault.

2. APPLICABILITY. This Directive:

a. Applies to:

(1) OSD, the Military Departments, the Office of the Chairman of the Joint Chiefs of Staff and the Joint Staff, the Combatant Commands, the Inspector General of the DoD (IG DoD), the Defense Agencies, the DoD Field Activities, and all other organizational entities within the DoD (hereafter referred to collectively as the "DoD Components").

(2) National Guard and Reserve Component members who are sexually assaulted when performing active service, as defined in section 101(d)(3) of Reference (b), and inactive duty training. Refer to DoD Instruction (DoDI) 6495.02 (Reference (c)) for additional SAPR and medical services provided to such personnel and eligibility criteria for Restricted Reporting.

(3) Military dependents 18 years of age and older who are eligible for treatment in the military healthcare system, at installations in the

continental United States (CONUS) and outside of the continental United States (OCONUS), and who were victims of sexual assault perpetrated by someone other than a spouse or intimate partner. The Family Advocacy Program (FAP) (DoDD 6400.1 (Reference (d))) provides the full range of services to victims of domestic violence who are sexually assaulted, in violation of Articles 120 (Rape and Sexual Assault) and 125 (Sodomy) of chapter 47 of Reference (b) (also known as and hereinafter referred to as "The Uniform Code of Military Justice (UCMJ)"), by someone with whom they have or have had an intimate partner relationship. The installation SARC and the installation family advocacy program (FAP) and domestic violence intervention and prevention staff shall direct coordination when a sexual assault occurs within a domestic relationship or involves child abuse.

(4) The following non–military personnel who are only eligible for LIMITED medical services in the form of emergency care (see Glossary), unless otherwise eligible to receive treatment in a military medical treatment facility. They will also be offered the LIMITED SAPR services of a Sexual Assault Response Coordinator (SARC) and a SAPR Victim Advocate (VA) while undergoing emergency care OCONUS. Refer to Reference (c) for any additional SAPR and medical services provided. These limited medical and SAPR services shall be provided to:

(a) DoD civilian employees and their family dependents 18 years of age and older when they are stationed or performing duties OCONUS and eligible for treatment in the military healthcare system at military installations or facilities OCONUS. Refer to Reference (c) for reporting options available to DoD civilians and their family dependents 18 years of age and older.

(b) U.S. citizen DoD contractor personnel when they are authorized to accompany the Armed Forces in a contingency operation OCONUS and their U.S. citizen employees (See DoDI 3020.41 (Reference (f))). Refer to Reference (c) for reporting options available to DoD contractors.

(5) Service members who are on active duty but were victims of sexual assault prior to enlistment or commissioning. They are eligible to receive full SAPR services and either reporting option.

b. Supersedes all policy and regulatory guidance within the DoD not expressly mandated by law that is inconsistent with its provisions, or that would preclude execution.

3. DEFINITIONS. See Glossary.

4. POLICY. It is DoD policy that:
a. This Directive and Reference (c) implement the DoD SAPR policy.
b. The DoD goal is a culture free of sexual assault, through an environment of prevention, education and training, response capability (defined in Reference (c)), victim support, reporting procedures, and appropriate accountability that enhances the safety and well being of all persons covered by this Directive and Reference (c).
c. The SAPR Program shall:
   (1) Focus on the victim and on doing what is necessary and appropriate to support victim recovery, and also, if a Service member, to support that Service member to be fully mission capable and engaged. The SAPR Program shall provide care that is gender-responsive, culturally-competent, and recovery-oriented (see Glossary).
   (2) NOT provide policy for legal processes within the responsibility of the Judge Advocates General of the Military Departments provided in Chapter 47 of Reference (b) and the Manual for Courts-Martial (Reference (g)) or for criminal investigative matters assigned to the IG DoD.

d. Standardized SAPR requirements, terminology, guidelines, protocols, and guidelines for instructional materials shall focus on awareness, prevention, and response at all levels as appropriate.
e. The terms "Sexual Assault Response Coordinator (SARC)" and "SAPR Victim Advocate (VA)," as defined in this Directive and the Reference (c), shall be used as standard terms throughout the DoD to facilitate communications and transparency regarding SAPR capacity. For further information regarding SARC and SAPR VA roles and responsibilities, see Reference (c).
   (1) SARC. The SARC shall serve as the SINGLE POINT OF CONTACT for coordinating appropriate and responsive care for sexual assault victims. SARCs shall coordinate sexual assault victim care and sexual assault response when a sexual assault is reported. The SARC

shall supervise SAPR VAs, but may be called on to perform victim advocacy duties.

(2) SAPR VA. The SAPR VA shall provide non–clinical crisis intervention and on–going support, in addition to referrals for adult sexual assault victims. Support will include providing information on available options and resources to victims.

f. Command sexual assault awareness and prevention programs, as well as law enforcement and criminal justice procedures that enable persons to be held accountable for their actions, as appropriate, shall be established and supported by all commanders.

g. An immediate, trained sexual assault response capability (defined in Reference (c)) shall be available for each report of sexual assault in all locations, including in deployed locations. The response time may be affected by operational necessities, but will reflect that sexual assault victims shall be treated as emergency cases.

h. Victims of sexual assault shall be protected from coercion, retaliation, and reprisal in accordance with DoDD 7050.06, (Reference (h)).

i. Victims of sexual assault shall be protected, treated with dignity and respect, and shall receive timely access to comprehensive medical treatment, including emergency care treatment and services, as described in this Directive and Reference (c).

j. Emergency care shall consist of emergency medical care and the offer of a sexual assault forensic examination (SAFE) consistent with the Department of Justice protocol (Reference (i)) and refer to DD Form 2911, "DoD Sexual Assault Medical Forensic Examination Report" and accompanying instructions. The victim shall be advised that even if a SAFE is declined, the victim is encouraged (but not mandated) to receive medical care, psychological care, and victim advocacy.

(1) Sexual assault patients shall be given priority, and shall be treated as emergency cases. A sexual assault victim needs immediate medical intervention to prevent loss of life or suffering resulting from physical injuries (internal or external), sexually transmitted infections, pregnancy, and psychological distress. Individuals disclosing a recent sexual assault shall, with their consent, be quickly transported to the exam site, promptly evaluated, treated for serious injuries, and then, with the patient's consent, undergo a SAFE, pursuant to "Victim Centered Care" of Reference (i) and refer to DD Form 2911 and accompanying instructions.

(2) Sexual assault patients shall be treated as emergency cases, regardless of whether physical injuries are evident. Patients' needs shall be assessed for immediate medical or mental health intervention pursuant to "Victim Centered Care," and "Triage and Intake" of Reference (i). Sexual assault victims shall be treated uniformly, consistent with "Victim Centered Care" of Reference (i) and DD Form 2911 and accompanying instructions, regardless of their behavior because when severely traumatized, sexual assault patients may appear to be calm, indifferent, submissive, jocular, angry, emotionally distraught, or even uncooperative or hostile towards those who are trying to help.

k. Service members and their dependents who are 18 years of age or older covered by this Directive (see subparagraph 2a.(4)) and Reference (c)) who are sexually assaulted have two reporting options: Unrestricted or Restricted Reporting. Complete, Unrestricted Reporting of sexual assault is favored by the DoD. See Reference (c) for additional information on the DoD sexual assault reporting options and exceptions as they apply to Restricted Reporting. Consult DoDD 5400.11 (Reference (j)) and DoD 6025.18-R (Reference (k)) for protections of personally identifiable information solicited, collected, maintained, accessed, used, disclosed, and disposed during the treatment and reporting processes. The two reporting options are as follows:

(1) Unrestricted Reporting allows an eligible person who is sexually assaulted to access medical treatment and counseling and request an official investigation of the allegation using existing reporting channels (e.g., chain of command, law enforcement, healthcare personnel, the SARC). When a sexual assault is reported through Unrestricted Reporting, a SARC shall be notified as soon as possible, respond, assign a SAPR VA, and offer the victim medical care and a SAFE.

(2) Restricted Reporting allows sexual assault victims (see eligibility criteria in Reference (c)) to confidentially disclose the assault to specified individuals (i.e., SARC, SAPR VA, or healthcare personnel), in accordance with Reference (j), and receive medical treatment, including emergency care, counseling, and assignment of a SARC and SAPR VA, without triggering an official investigation. The victim's report to healthcare personnel (including the information acquired from a SAFE Kit), SARCs, or SAPR VAs will NOT be reported to law enforcement or to the victim's

command, to initiate the official investigative process, unless the victim consents or an established EXCEPTION applies in accordance with Reference (c). When a sexual assault is reported through Restricted Reporting, a SARC shall be notified as soon as possible, respond, assign a SAPR VA, and offer the victim medical care and a SAFE.

(a) Eligibility for Restricted Reporting. The Restricted Reporting Program applies to Service members and their military dependents 18 years of age and older. For additional persons who may be entitled to Restricted Reporting, see eligibility criteria in Reference (c).

(b) DoD Dual Objectives. The DoD is committed to ensuring victims of sexual assault are protected; treated with dignity and respect; and provided support, advocacy, and care. The DoD supports effective command awareness and prevention programs. The DoD also strongly supports applicable law enforcement and criminal justice procedures that enable persons to be held accountable for sexual assault offenses and criminal dispositions, as appropriate. To achieve these dual objectives, DoD preference is for complete Unrestricted Reporting of sexual assaults to allow for the provision of victims' services and to pursue accountability. However, Unrestricted Reporting may represent a barrier for victims to access services, when the victim desires no command or law enforcement involvement. Consequently, the DoD recognizes a fundamental need to provide a confidential disclosure vehicle via the Restricted Reporting option.

(c) Designated Personnel Authorized to Accept a Restricted Report. Only the SARC, SAPR VA, or healthcare personnel are designated as authorized to accept a Restricted Report.

(d) SAFE Confidentiality Under Restricted Reporting. A SAFE and its information shall be afforded the same confidentiality as is afforded victim statements under the Restricted Reporting option. See Reference (c) for additional information.

(e) Disclosure of Confidential Communications. In cases where a victim elects Restricted Reporting, the SARC, assigned SAPR VA, and healthcare personnel may not disclose confidential communications or SAFE Kit information to law enforcement or command authorities, either within or outside the DoD, EXCEPT as provided in Reference (c). In certain situations when information about a sexual assault comes to the commander's or law enforcement official's attention from a source independent of the Restricted Reporting avenues and an independent investigation is initiated, a SARC, SAPR VA, or healthcare personnel may NOT disclose confidential communications if obtained under Restricted Reporting (see exceptions to Restricted Reporting in Reference (c)). Improper disclosure of confidential communications under Restricted Reporting, improper release of medical information, and other violations of this policy are prohibited and may result in discipline pursuant to the UCMJ, or other adverse personnel or administrative actions.

l. Enlistment or commissioning of personnel in the Military Services shall be prohibited and no waivers are allowed when the person has a qualifying conviction (see Glossary) for a crime of sexual assault.
m. The focus of this Directive and Reference (c) is on the victim of sexual assault. The DoD shall provide support to an active duty Service member regardless of when or where the sexual assault took place.

5. RESPONSIBILITIES. See Enclosure 2.

6. INFORMATION COLLECTION REQUIREMENTS
   a. The sexual assault reporting requirements in this Directive have been assigned Report Control Symbol (RCS) DD-P&R(A) 2205 in accordance with DoD 8910.1-M (Reference (l)).
   b. The Defense Sexual Assault Incident Database (DSAID) information collection referred to in paragraphs 1f, 6l, 6n, and 6o of Enclosure 2 of this directive is submitted to Congress in accordance with sections 561, 562, and 563 of Public Law 110-417 (Reference (p)) and is coordinated with the Assistant Secretary of Defense for Legislative Affairs in accordance with the procedures in DoD Instruction 5545.02 (Reference (t)).

7. RELEASABILITY. UNLIMITED. This Directive is approved for public release and is available on the Internet from the DoD Issuances Website at http://www.dtic.mil/whs/directives.

8. EFFECTIVE DATE. This Directive:
   a. Is effective January 23, 2012.
   b. Must be reissued, cancelled, or certified current within 5 years of its publication in accordance with DoDI 5025.01 (Reference (e)). If not, it will expire effective January 23, 2022 and be removed from the DoD Issuances Website.

ENCLOSURE 1

REFERENCES

  (a) DoD Directive 6495.01, "Sexual Assault Prevention and Response (SAPR) Program," October 6, 2005 (hereby cancelled)

  (b) Sections 101(d)(3) and 113, chapter 47,1 and chapter 80 of title 10, United States Code

  (c) DoD Instruction 6495.02, "Sexual Assault Prevention and Response Program Procedures," November 13, 2008

  (d) DoD Directive 6400.1, "Family Advocacy Program (FAP)," August 23, 2004

  (e) DoD Instruction 5025.01, "DoD Directives Program," September 26, 2012

  (f) DoD Instruction 3020.41, "Operational Contract Support (OCS)," December 20, 2011

  (g) U.S. Department of Defense, "Manual for Courts-Martial," 2008

  (h) DoD Directive 7050.06, "Military Whistleblower Protection," July 23, 2007

  (i) U.S. Department of Justice, Office on Violence Against Women, "A National Protocol for Sexual Assault Medical Forensic Examinations, Adults/Adolescents," current version

  (j) DoD Directive 5400.11, "DoD Privacy Program," May 8, 2007

  (k) DoD 6025.18-R, "DoD Health Information Privacy Regulation," January 24, 2003

  (l) DoD 8910.1-M, "DoD Procedures for Management of Information Requirements," June 30, 1998

  (m)DoD Directive 5124.02, "Under Secretary of Defense for Personnel and Readiness (USD(P&R))," June 23, 2008

  (n) U.S. Department of Defense Paper, "The Department of Defense Sexual Assault Prevention Strategy," September 30, 2008

  (o) Section 577 of Public Law 108-375, "Ronald Reagan National Defense Authorization Act for Fiscal Year 2005," October 28, 2004

  (p) Sections 561, 562, and 563 of Public Law 110-417, "The Duncan Hunter National Defense Authorization Act for Fiscal Year 2009," October 14, 2008

  (q) Section 567(c) of Public Law 111-84, "The National Defense Authorization Act for Fiscal Year 2010," October 28, 2009

  (r) Joint Publication 1-02, "Department of Defense Dictionary of Military and Associated Terms," current edition

(s) DoD Instruction 5545.02, "DoD Policy for Congressional Authorization and Appropriations Reporting Requirement," December 19, 2008

ENCLOSURE 2
RESPONSIBILITIES

1. UNDER SECRETARY OF DEFENSE FOR PERSONNEL AND READINESS (USD(P&R)). In accordance with the authority in DoDD 5124.02 (Reference (m)), the USD(P&R) shall:

   a. Develop overall policy and provide oversight for the DoD SAPR Program, except legal processes in the UCMJ and criminal investigative matters assigned to the Judge Advocates General of the Military Departments and IG DoD, respectively.

   b. Develop strategic program guidance, joint planning objectives, standard terminology, and identify legislative changes needed to ensure the future availability of resources in support of DoD SAPR policies.

   c. Develop metrics to measure compliance and effectiveness of SAPR training, awareness, prevention, and response policies and programs. Analyze data and make recommendations regarding the SAPR policies and programs to the Secretaries of the Military Departments.

   d. Monitor compliance with this Directive and Reference (c), and coordinate with the Secretaries of the Military Departments regarding Service SAPR policies.

   e. Collaborate with Federal and State agencies that address SAPR issues and serve as liaison to them as appropriate. Strengthen collaboration on sexual assault policy matters with U.S. Department of Veterans Affairs on the issues of providing high quality and accessible health care and benefits to victims of sexual assault.

   f. Oversee the DoD Sexual Assault Prevention and Response Office (SAPRO). Serving as the DoD single point of authority, accountability, and oversight for the SAPR program, SAPRO provides recommendations to the USD(P&R) on the issue of DoD sexual assault policy matters on prevention, response, and oversight. SAPRO is responsible for:

   (1) Implementing and monitoring compliance with DoD sexual assault policy on prevention and response, except for legal processes in the UCMJ and Reference (g), and criminal investigative matters assigned to the Judge Advocate General of the Military Departments and IG DoD, respectively.

(2) Providing technical assistance to the Heads of the DoD Components in addressing matters concerning SAPR.

(3) Acquiring quarterly and annual SAPR data from the Military Services, assembling annual congressional reports involving persons covered by this Directive and Reference (c), and consulting with and relying on the Judge Advocate General of the Military Departments in questions concerning disposition results of sexual assault cases in their respective departments.

(4) Establishing reporting categories and monitor specific goals included in the annual SAPR assessments of each Military Service, in their respective departments.

(5) Overseeing the creation, implementation, maintenance, and function of the DSAID, an integrated database that will meet congressional reporting requirements, support Service SAPR Program management, and inform DoD SAPRO oversight activities.

2. ASSISTANT SECRETARY OF DEFENSE FOR HEALTH AFFAIRS (ASD(HA)). The ASD(HA), under the authority, direction, and control of the USD(P&R), shall advise the USD(P&R) on DoD sexual assault healthcare policies, clinical practice guidelines, related procedures, and standards governing DoD healthcare programs for victims of sexual assault. The ASD(HA) shall direct that all sexual assault patients be given priority, so that they shall be treated as emergency cases.

3. DIRECTOR, DEPARTMENT OF DEFENSE HUMAN RESOURCES ACTIVITY (DoDHRA). The Director of DoDHRA, under the authority, direction, and control of USD(P&R), shall provide operational support to the USD(P&R) as outlined in paragraph 1.f. of this enclosure.

4. GENERAL COUNSEL OF THE DoD (GC, DoD). The GC, DoD, shall provide legal advice and assistance on all legal matters, including the review and coordination of all proposed issuances and exceptions to policy and the review of all legislative proposals, affecting mission and responsibilities of the DoD SAPRO.

5. IG DoD. The IG DoD shall:

a. Develop and oversee the promulgation of criminal investigative and law enforcement policy regarding sexual assault and establish guidelines for the collection and preservation of evidence with non-identifiable personal information on the victim, for the Restricted Reporting process, in coordination with the ASD(HA).

b. Oversee criminal investigations of sexual assault conducted by the DoD Components.

c. Collaborate with the DoD SAPRO in the development of investigative policy in support of sexual assault prevention and response.

6. SECRETARIES OF THE MILITARY DEPARTMENTS. The Secretaries of the Military Departments shall:

a. Establish departmental policies and procedures to implement the SAPR Program consistent with the provisions of this Directive and Reference (c), to include the military academies within their cognizance; monitor departmental compliance with this Directive and Reference (c).

b. Coordinate all Military Service SAPR policy changes with the USD(P&R).

c. In coordination with the USD(P&R), implement recommendations regarding Military Service compliance and effectiveness of SAPR training, awareness, prevention, and response policies and programs.

d. Align Service SAPR strategic plans with the DoD SAPR strategic plan.

e. Align Service prevention strategy with the Spectrum of Prevention consistent with the DoD Sexual Assault Prevention Strategy (Reference (n)), which consists of six pillars:

(1) Influencing Policy

(2) Changing Organizational Practices

(3) Fostering Coalitions and Networks

(4) Educating Providers

(5) Promoting Community Education

(6) Strengthening Individual Knowledge and Skills

f. Require commanders to ensure that medical treatment (including emergency care) and SAPR services are provided to victims of sexual assaults in a timely manner unless declined by the victim.

g. Utilize the terms "Sexual Assault Response Coordinator (SARC)" and "SAPR Victim Advocate (VA)," as defined in this Directive and Reference (c), as standard terms to facilitate communications and transparency regarding sexual assault response capacity.

h. Establish the position of the SARC to serve as the SINGLE POINT OF CONTACT for ensuring that sexual assault victims receive appropriate and responsive care. The SARC should be a Service member, DoD civilian employee, or National Guard technician.

i. Provide program-appropriate resources to enable the Combatant Commanders to achieve compliance with the policies set forth in this Directive and Reference (c).

j. Establish and codify Service SAPR Program support to Combatant Commands and Defense Agencies, either as a host activity or in a deployed environment.

k. Provide SAPR Program and obligation data to the USD(P&R), as required.

l. Submit quarterly reports to the USD(P&R) that include information regarding all sexual assaults reported during the quarter, until DSAID becomes fully operational for each individual Service. Require confirmation that a multi-disciplinary case management group tracks each open Unrestricted Report and that a multi-disciplinary case management group meetings are held monthly for reviewing all Unrestricted Reports of sexual assaults.

m. Provide annual reports of sexual assaults involving persons covered by this Directive and Reference (c) to the DoD SAPRO for consolidation into the annual report to Congress in accordance with section 577 of Public Law 108-375 (Reference (o)).

n. Provide data connectivity, or other means, to authorized users to ensure all sexual assaults reported in theater and other joint environments are incorporated into the DSAID, or authorized interfacing systems for the documentation of reports of sexual assault, as required by section 563 of Public Law 110-417 (Reference (p)).

o. Ensure that Service data systems used to report case-level sexual assault information into the DSAID are compliant with DoD data reporting requirements, pursuant to section 563 of Reference (p).

p. Require extensive, continuing in-depth SAPR training for DoD personnel and specialized SAPR training for commanders, senior enlisted leaders, SARCs, SAPR VAs, investigators, law enforcement officials, chaplains, healthcare personnel, and legal personnel in accordance with Reference (c).

q. Oversee sexual assault training within the DoD law enforcement community.

r. Direct that Service military criminal investigative organizations require their investigative units to communicate with their servicing SARC and participate with the multi-disciplinary Case Management Group convened by the SARC, in accordance with this Directive and Reference (c).

s. Provide commanders with procedures that:

(1) Establish guidance for when a Military Protective Order (MPO) has been issued, that the Service member who is protected by the order is informed, in a timely manner, of the member's option to request transfer from the command to which that member is assigned in accordance with section 567(c) of Public Law 111-84 (Reference (q)).

(2) Ensure that the appropriate civilian authorities shall be notified of the issuance of a MPO and of the individuals involved in the order, when an MPO has been issued against a Service member or when any individual addressed in the MPO does not reside on a military installation at any time when an MPO is in effect. An MPO issued by a military commander shall remain in effect until such time as the commander terminates the order or issues a replacement order. (See section 561 of Reference (p).) The issuing commander also shall notify the appropriate civilian authorities of any change made in a protective order covered by chapter 80 of Reference (b), and the termination of the protective order.

(3) Ensure that the person seeking the MPO shall be advised that the MPO is not enforceable by civilian authorities off base and that victims desiring protection off base are advised to seek a civilian protective order. (See section 561 of Reference (p) and section 567 of Reference (q).)

7. CHAIRMAN OF THE JOINT CHIEFS OF STAFF. The Chairman of the Joint Chiefs of Staff shall:

   a. Assess SAPR as part of the overall force planning function of any force deployment decision, and periodically reassess the SAPR posture of deployed forces.

   b. Monitor implementation of this Directive, Reference (c), and implementing instructions, including during military operations.

   c. Utilize the terms "Sexual Assault Response Coordinator (SARC)" and "SAPR Victim Advocate (VA)," as defined in this Directive and Reference (c), as standard terms to facilitate communications and transparency regarding sexual assault response capacity.

   d. Review relevant documents, including the Combatant Commanders' joint plans, operational plans, concept plans, and deployment orders, to ensure they identify and include SAPR Program requirements.

8. COMMANDERS OF THE COMBATANT COMMANDS. The Commanders of the Combatant Commands, in coordination with the other Heads of the DoD Components and through the Chairman of the Joint Chiefs of Staff, shall:

a. Establish policies and procedures to implement the SAPR Program and oversee compliance with this Directive and Reference (c) within their areas of responsibility and during military operations.

b. Formally document agreements with installation host Service commanders, component theater commanders, or other heads of another agency or organization, for investigative, legal, medical, counseling, or other response support provided to incidents of sexual assault.

c. Direct that relevant documents are drafted, including joint operational plans and deployment orders, that establish theater-level requirements for the prevention of and response to incidents of sexual assault that occur, to include during the time of military operations.

d. Require that sexual assault response capability information be provided to all persons within their area of responsibility covered by this Directive and Reference (c), to include reporting options and SAPR services available at deployed locations and how to access these options.

e. Ensure medical treatment (including emergency care) and SAPR services are provided to victims of sexual assaults in a timely manner unless declined by the victim.

f. Direct subordinate commanders coordinate relationships and agreements for host or installation support at forward–deployed locations to ensure a sexual assault response capability is available to members of their command and persons covered by this Directive and Reference (c) as consistent with operational requirements.

g. Direct that sexual assault incidents are given priority so that they shall be treated as emergency cases.

h. Direct [that] subordinate commanders provide all personnel with procedures to report sexual assaults.

i. Require subordinate commanders at all levels to monitor the command climate with respect to SAPR, and take appropriate steps to address problems.

j. Require that SAPR training for DoD personnel and specialized training for commanders, senior enlisted leaders, SARCs, SAPR VAs, investigators, law enforcement officials, chaplains, healthcare personnel, and legal personnel be conducted prior to deployment in accordance with Reference (c).

k. Direct subordinate commanders to develop procedures that:

(1) Establish guidance for when an MPO has been issued, that the Service member who is protected by the order is informed, in a timely manner, of the member's option to request transfer from the command to which that member is assigned in accordance with section 567(c) of Reference (q).

(2) In OCONUS areas, if appropriate, direct that the appropriate civilian authorities be notified of the issuance of an MPO and of the individuals involved in an order when an MPO has been issued against a Service member or when any individual involved in the MPO does not reside on a military installation when an MPO is in effect. An MPO issued by a military commander shall remain in effect until such time as the commander terminates the order or issues a replacement order. (See section 561 of Reference (p).) The issuing commander also shall notify the appropriate civilian authorities of any change made in a protective order covered by chapter 80 of Reference (b) and the termination of the protective order.

(3) Ensure that the person seeking the MPO is advised that the MPO is not enforceable by civilian authorities off base, and victims desiring protection off base should be advised to seek a civilian protective order in that jurisdiction pursuant to section 562 of Reference (p).

Table 7.1. Glossary

PART I. ABBREVIATIONS AND ACRONYMS	
ASD(HA)	Assistant Secretary of Defense for Health Affairs
CONUS	Continental United States
DoDD	Department of Defense Directive
DoDHRA	Department of Defense Human Resources Activity
DoDI	Department of Defense Instruction
DSAID	Defense Sexual Assault Incident Database
FAP	Family Advocacy Program
IG DoD	Inspector General of the Department of Defense
GC, DoD	General Counsel of the Department of Defense
MPO	Military Protective Order
OCONUS	outside of the continental United States
SAFE	sexual assault forensic examination
SAPR	sexual assault prevention and response
SAPR VA	Sexual Assault Prevention and Response Victim Advocate
SAPRO	Sexual Assault Prevention and Response Office
SARC	Sexual Assault Response Coordinator
UCMJ	Uniform Code of Military Justice
U.S.C.	United States Code
USD(P&R)	Under Secretary of Defense for Personnel and Readiness

PART II. DEFINITIONS

Unless otherwise noted, these terms and their definitions are for the purpose of this Directive.

confidential communication. Oral, written, or electronic communications of personally identifiable information concerning a sexual assault victim and the sexual assault incident provided by the victim to the SARC, SAPR VA, or healthcare personnel in a Restricted Report. This confidential communication includes the victim's SAFE Kit and its information. See http://www.archives.gov/cui.

consent. Words or overt acts indicating a freely given agreement to the sexual conduct at issue by a competent person. An expression of lack of consent through words or conduct means there is no consent. Lack of verbal or physical resistance or submission resulting from the accused's use of force, threat of force, or placing another person in fear does not constitute consent. A current or previous dating relationship or the manner of dress of the person involved with the accused in the sexual conduct at issue shall not constitute consent. There is no consent where the person is sleeping or incapacitated, such as due to age, alcohol or drugs, or mental incapacity.

crisis intervention. Emergency non–clinical care aimed at assisting victims in alleviating potential negative consequences by providing safety assessments and connecting victims to needed resources. Either the SARC or SAPR VA will intervene as quickly as possible to assess the victim's safety and determine the needs of victims and connect them to appropriate referrals, as needed.

culturally-competent care. Care that provides culturally and linguistically appropriate services.

DSAID. A DoD database that captures uniform data provided by the Military Services and maintains all sexual assault data collected by the Military Services. This database shall be a centralized, case-level database for the uniform collection of data regarding incidence of sexual assaults involving persons covered by this Directive and Reference (c). DSAID will include information when available, or when not limited by Restricted Reporting, or otherwise prohibited by law, about the nature of the assault, the victim, the offender, and the disposition of reports associated with the assault. DSAID shall be available to the SAPRO and the DoD to develop and implement congressional reporting requirements. Unless authorized by law, or needed for internal DoD review or analysis, disclosure of data stored in DSAID will only be granted when disclosure is ordered by a military, Federal, or State judge or other officials or entities as required by a law or applicable U.S. international agreement. This term and its definition are proposed for inclusion in the next edition of Joint Publication 1-02 (Reference [r]).

emergency. A situation that requires immediate intervention to prevent the loss of life, limb, sight, or body tissue to prevent undue suffering. Regardless of appearance, a sexual assault victim needs immediate medical intervention to prevent loss of life or undue suffering resulting from physical injuries internal or external, sexually transmitted infections, pregnancy, or psychological distress. Sexual assault victims shall be given priority as emergency cases regardless of evidence of physical injury.

emergency care. Emergency medical care includes physical and emergency psychological medical services and a SAFE consistent with Reference (i).

gender-responsive care. Care that acknowledges and is sensitive to gender differences and gender-specific issues.

healthcare personnel. Persons assisting or otherwise supporting healthcare providers in providing healthcare services (e.g., administrative personnel assigned to a military medical treatment facility, or mental healthcare personnel). Healthcare personnel also includes all healthcare providers.

Military Services. The term, as used in the SAPR Program, includes Army, Air Force, Navy, Marines, Reserve Components, and their respective Military Academies.

non-identifiable personal information. Non-identifiable personal information includes those facts and circumstances surrounding the sexual assault incident or that information about the individual that enables the identity of the individual to remain anonymous. In contrast, personal identifying information is information belonging to the victim and alleged assailant of a sexual assault that would disclose or have a tendency to disclose the person's identity.

official investigative process. The formal process a commander or law enforcement organization uses to gather evidence and examine the circumstances surrounding a report of sexual assault.

personal identifiable information. Includes the person's name, other particularly identifying descriptions (e.g., physical characteristics or identity by position, rank, or organization), or other information about the person or the facts and circumstances involved that could reasonably be understood to identify the person (e.g., a female in a particular squadron or barracks when there is only one female assigned).

qualifying conviction. A State or Federal conviction, or a finding of guilty in a juvenile adjudication, for a felony crime of sexual assault and any general or special court-martial conviction for a UCMJ offense, which otherwise meets the elements of a crime of sexual assault, even though not classified as a felony or misdemeanor within the UCMJ. In addition, any offense that requires registration as a sex offender is a qualifying conviction.

recovery-oriented care. Focus on the victim and on doing what is necessary and appropriate to support victim recovery, and also, if a Service member, to support that Service member to be fully mission capable and engaged.

Restricted Reporting. Reporting option that allows sexual assault victims to confidentially disclose the assault to specified individuals (i.e., SARC, SAPR VA, or healthcare personnel), in accordance with Reference (i), and receive medical treatment, including emergency care, counseling, and assignment of a SARC and SAPR VA, without triggering an official investigation. The victim's report provided to healthcare personnel (including the information acquired from a SAFE Kit), SARCs, or SAPR VAs will NOT be reported to law enforcement or to the command to initiate the official investigative process unless the victim consents or an established EXCEPTION applies in accordance with Reference (c). The Restricted Reporting Program applies to Service members and their military dependents 18 years of age and older. For additional persons who may be entitled to Restricted Reporting, see eligibility criteria in Reference (c). Only a SARC, SAPR VA, or healthcare personnel may receive a Restricted Report, previously referred to as Confidential Reporting. This term and its definition are proposed for inclusion in the next edition of Reference (r).

SAFE Kit. The medical and forensic examination of a sexual assault victim under circumstances and controlled procedures to ensure the physical examination process and the collection, handling, analysis, testing, and safekeeping of any bodily specimens and evidence meet the requirements necessary for use as evidence in criminal proceedings. The victim's SAFE Kit is treated as a confidential communication when conducted as part of a Restricted Report. This term and its definition are proposed for inclusion in the next edition of Reference (r).

SAPRO. Serves as the DoD's single point of authority, accountability, and oversight for the SAPR program, except for legal processes and criminal investigative matters that are the responsibility of the Judge Advocates General of the Military Departments and the IG, respectively. This term and its definition are proposed for inclusion in the next edition of Reference (r).

SAPR Program. A DoD program for the Military Departments and the DoD Components that establishes SAPR policies to be implemented worldwide. The program objective is an environment and military community intolerant of sexual assault. This term and its definition are proposed for inclusion in the next edition of Reference (r).

SAPR VA. A person who, as a victim advocate, shall provide non-clinical crisis intervention, referral, and ongoing non-clinical support to adult sexual assault victims. Support will include providing information on available options and resources to victims. The SAPR VA, on behalf of the sexual assault victim, provides liaison assistance with other organizations and agencies on victim care matters and reports directly to the SARC when performing victim advocacy duties. Personnel who are interested in serving as a SAPR VA are encouraged to volunteer for this duty assignment. This term and its definition are proposed for inclusion in the next edition of Reference (r).

SARC. The single point of contact at an installation or within a geographic area who oversees sexual assault awareness, prevention, and response training; coordinates medical treatment, including emergency care, for victims of sexual assault; and tracks the services provided to a victim of sexual assault from the initial report through final disposition and resolution. This term and its definition are proposed for inclusion in the next edition of Reference (r).

senior commander. An officer, usually in the grade of O-6 or higher, who is the commander of a military installation or comparable unit and has been designated by the Military Service concerned to oversee the SAPR Program.

Service member. An active duty member of a Military Service. In addition, National Guard and Reserve Component members who are sexually assaulted when performing active service, as defined in section 101(d)(3) of Reference (b), and inactive duty training.

sexual assault. Intentional sexual contact characterized by use of force, threats, intimidation, or abuse of authority or when the victim does not or cannot consent. The term includes a broad category of sexual offenses consisting of the following specific UCMJ offenses: rape, sexual assault, aggravated sexual contact, abusive sexual contact, forcible sodomy (forced oral or anal sex), or attempts to commit these acts.

Unrestricted Reporting. A process that an individual covered by this policy uses to disclose, without requesting confidentiality or Restricted Reporting, that he or she is the victim of a sexual assault. Under these circumstances, the victim's report provided to healthcare personnel, the SARC, a SAPR VA, command authorities, or other persons is reported to law enforcement and may be used to initiate the official investigative process. Additional policy and guidance are provided in Reference (c).

This term and its definition are proposed for inclusion in the next edition of Reference (r).

victim. A person who asserts direct physical, emotional, or pecuniary harm as a result of the commission of a sexual assault. The term encompasses all persons 18 and over eligible to receive treatment in military medical treatment facilities; however, the Restricted Reporting Program applies to Service members and their military dependents 18 years of age and older. For additional persons who may be entitled to Restricted Reporting, see eligibility criteria in Reference (c).

SEXUAL ASSAULT PREVENTION AND RESPONSE OFFICE (SAPRO)

SAPRO is the organization responsible for the oversight of Department of Defense (DoD) sexual assault policy. The Department of Defense is committed to the prevention of sexual assault. The Department has implemented a comprehensive policy to ensure the safety, dignity, and well-being of all members of the Armed Forces. Our men and women serving throughout the world deserve nothing less, and their leaders—both Military and civilian—are committed to maintaining a workplace environment that rejects sexual assault and reinforces a culture of prevention, response, and accountability.

Vision Statement

To enable military readiness by establishing a culture free of sexual assault

Mission

The Sexual Assault Prevention and Response Office will serve as the single point of accountability and oversight for sexual assault policy, provide guidance to the DoD components, and facilitate the resolution of issues common to all Military Services and joint commands.

The objectives of DoD's Sexual Assault Prevention and Response policy are to specifically enhance and improve:

Prevention through training and education programs
Treatment and support of victims
System accountability

Background

In February of 2004, former Secretary of Defense Donald H. Rumsfeld directed Dr. David S. C. Chu, former Under Secretary of Defense for Personnel and Readiness, to review the DoD process for treatment and care of victims of sexual assault in the Military Services (www.sapr.mil/public/docs/laws/d20040213satf.pdf).

The Department quickly assembled the Care for Victims of Sexual Assault Task Force, led by Ms. Ellen Embrey, Deputy Assistant Secretary of Defense for Force Health, Protection, and Readiness, and charged the task force to report back in 90 days with recommendations (Task Force Report for Care of Victims of SA, www.sapr.mil/public/docs/reports/task-force-report-for-care-of-victims-of-sa-2004.pdf). Following a comprehensive review, the Task Force released a series of recommendations in April 2004.

One of the recommendations emphasized the need to establish a single point of accountability for sexual assault policy within the Department. This led to the establishment of the Joint Task Force for Sexual Assault Prevention and Response, and the naming of then Brigadier General K.C. McClain as its commander in October 2004. The Task Force focused its initial efforts on developing a new DoD-wide sexual assault policy that incorporated recommendations set forth in the Task Force Report on Care for Victims of Sexual Assault as well as in the Ronald W. Reagan National Defense Authorization Act for Fiscal Year 2005 (PL108-375). This act directed the Department to have a sexual assault policy in place by January 1, 2005. In January 2005, DoD presented to Congress a comprehensive policy on prevention and response to sexual assault. The policy provides a foundation for the Department to improve prevention of sexual assault, significantly enhance support to victims, and increase reporting and accountability.

The Task Force and the Military Services collaborated closely to ensure the rapid and effective implementation of this policy. In 2005, the Task Force provided instruction to more than 1,200 sexual assault response coordinators (SARCs), chaplains, lawyers, and law enforcement to create a cadre of trained first responders. In addition, the Military Services trained more than 1,000,000 Service members and established sexual assault program offices at all major installations. The overarching elements of sexual assault prevention and response policy became permanent with the approval of DoD Directive 6495.01 (www.sapr.mil/public/docs/directives/649501p.pdf), Sexual Assault Prevention and Response Policy, in October 2005. The Task Force began transitioning into a permanent office that same month.

The Sexual Assault Prevention and Response Office (SAPRO) now serves as the Department's single point of authority for sexual assault policy and provides oversight to ensure that each of the Services' programs complies with DoD policy. It quickly obtained approval of DoD Instruction 6495.02 (http://www.dtic.mil/whs/directives/corres/pdf/649502p.pdf), Sexual Assault Prevention and Response Program Procedures, making permanent all elements of the Department's sexual assault policy. In addition, it conducted a training conference for all SARCs.

SAPRO, under the leadership of Major General Gary S. Patton (http://www.defense.gov/news/PattonBiography.pdf), continues to lead the Department's effort to transform into action its commitment to sexual assault prevention and response. This undertaking enjoys the support of leaders at all levels, and it will create a climate of confidence and trust where everyone is afforded respect and dignity.

Responsibilities

1. UNDER SECRETARY OF DEFENSE FOR PERSONNEL AND READINESS (USD(P&R)). The USD(P&R), in accordance with the authority in References (a) and (b), shall:
   a. Oversee the DoD Sexual Assault Prevention and Response Office (SAPRO) (see Glossary in Reference (b)) in accordance with Reference (b).
   b. Direct DoD Component implementation of this Instruction in compliance with Reference (b).
   c. Direct that Director, SAPRO, be informed of and consulted on any changes in DoD policy or the UCMJ relating to sexual assault.
   d. With the Director, SAPRO, update the Deputy Secretary of Defense on SAPR policies and programs on a semi-annual schedule.
   e. Direct the creation, implementation, and maintenance of DSAID.
   f. Oversee DoD SAPRO in developing DoD requirements for SAPR education, training, and awareness for DoD personnel consistent with this Instruction.
   g. Appoint a general or flag officer (G/FO) or Senior Executive Service (SES) equivalent in the DoD as the Director, SAPRO.
   h. In addition to the Director, SAPRO, assign a military officer from each of the Military Services in the grade of O–4 or above to SAPRO for a minimum tour length of at least 18 months. Of these four officers assigned to the SAPRO, at least one officer shall be in the grade of O–6 or above. See Reference (l).

i. Establish a DoD-wide certification program (see Glossary) with a national accreditor to ensure all sexual assault victims are offered the assistance of a SARC or SAPR VA who has obtained this certification.

2. DIRECTOR, DEPARTMENT OF DEFENSE HUMAN RESOURCE ACTIVITY (DoDHRA). The Director, DoDHRA, under the authority, direction, and control of the USD(P&R), shall provide operational support, budget, and allocate funds and other resources for the DoD SAPRO as outlined in Reference (b).

a. Establish DoD sexual assault healthcare policies, clinical practice guidelines, related procedures, and standards governing the DoD healthcare programs for victims of sexual assault.

b. Oversee the requirements and procedures in Enclosure 7 of this Instruction.

c. Establish guidance to:

(1) Give priority to sexual assault patients at MTFs as emergency cases.

(2) Require standardized, timely, accessible, and comprehensive medical care at MTFs for eligible persons who are sexually assaulted.

(3) Require that medical care is consistent with established community standards for the healthcare of sexual assault victims and the collection of forensic evidence from victims, in accordance with the U.S. Department of Justice Protocol (Reference (w)), instructions for victim and suspect exams found in the SAFE Kit, and DD Form 2911.

(a) Minimum standards of healthcare intervention that correspond to clinical standards set in the community shall include those established in Reference (w). However, clinical guidance shall not be solely limited to this resource.

(b) Healthcare providers providing care to sexual assault victims in theaters of operation are required to have access to the current version of Reference (w).

(4) Include deliberate planning to strategically position healthcare providers skilled in SAFE at predetermined echelons of care, for personnel with the responsibility of assigning medical assets.

d. Establish guidance for medical personnel that requires a SARC or SAPR VA to be called in for every incident of sexual assault for which treatment is sought at the MTFs, regardless of the reporting option.

e. Establish guidance in drafting memorandums of understanding (MOUs) or memorandums of agreement (MOAs) with local civilian medical facilities to provide DoD-reimbursable healthcare (to include psychological care) and forensic examinations for Service members and TRICARE eligible sexual assault victims.

    (1) As part of the MOU or MOA, victims shall be asked whether they would like the SARC to be notified and, if notified, a SARC or SAPR VA shall respond.

    (2) Local private or public sector providers shall have processes and procedures in place to assess that local community standards meet or exceed the recommendations for conducting forensic exams of adult sexual assault victims set forth in Reference (w) as a condition of the MOUs or MOAs.

f. Establish guidelines and procedures for the Surgeons General of the Military Departments to require that an adequate supply of resources, to include personnel, supplies, and SAFE Kits, is maintained in all locations where SAFEs may be conducted by DoD, including deployed locations. Maintaining an adequate supply of SAFE Kits is a shared responsibility of the ASD(HA) and Secretaries of the Military Departments.

g. Establish minimum standards of initial and refresher SAPR training required for all personnel assigned to MTFs. Specialized responder training is required for personnel providing direct care to victims of sexual assault. Minimum standards shall include trauma-informed care (see Glossary) and medical and mental health care that is gender-responsive, culturally-competent, and recovery-oriented.

4. GENERAL COUNSEL OF THE DEPARTMENT OF DEFENSE (GC, DoD). The GC, DoD, shall:

a. Provide legal advice and assistance on proposed policies, DoD issuances, proposed exceptions to policy, and review of all legislative proposals affecting mission and responsibilities of the Sexual Assault Prevention and Response Office.

b. Inform the USD(P&R) of any sexual assault related changes to the UCMJ.

5. IG DOD. The IG DoD, shall:

a. Establish guidance and provide oversight for the investigations of sexual assault in the DoD to meet the SAPR policy and training requirements of this Instruction.

b. Inform the USD(P&R) of any changes relating to sexual assault investigation policy or guidance.

c. Collaborate with SAPRO in the development of investigative policy in support of sexual assault prevention and response.

6. SECRETARIES OF THE MILITARY DEPARTMENTS. The Secretaries of the Military Departments shall:

a. Establish SAPR policy and procedures to implement this Instruction.

b. Coordinate all Military Service SAPR policy changes (Department of the Navy-level for the Navy and Marine Corps) with the USD(P&R).

c. Establish and publicize policies and procedures regarding the availability of a SARC.

   (1) Require that sexual assault victims receive appropriate and responsive care and that the SARC serves as the single point of contact for coordinating care for victims.

   (2) Direct that the SARC or a SAPR VA be immediately called in every incident of sexual assault on a military installation. There will be situations where a sexual assault victim receives medical care and a SAFE outside of a military installation through an MOU or MOA with a local private or public sector entity. In these cases, the MOU or MOA will require that victims shall be asked whether they would like the SARC to be notified as part of the MOU or MOA, and, if yes, a SARC or VA shall be notified and shall respond.

   (3) When a victim has a temporary change of station or permanent change of station or is deployed, direct that SARCs immediately request victim consent in writing to transfer case management documents, which should be documented on the DD Form 2910. Upon receipt of victim consent, SARCs shall expeditiously transfer case management documents to ensure continuity of care and SAPR services. All Federal, DoD, and Service privacy regulations must be strictly adhered to. However, when the SARC has a temporary change of station or permanent change of station or is deployed, no victim consent is required to transfer the case to the next SARC. Every effort must be made to inform the victim of the case transfer. If the SARC has already closed the case and terminated victim contact, no other action is needed.

    (4) Upon the full implementation of the DoD Sexual Assault Advocate Certification Program (D-SAACP), sexual assault victims shall be offered the assistance of a SARC and/or SAPR VA who has been credentialed by the D-SAACP and has passed a National Agency Check (NAC) background check.

    (5) Issue guidance to ensure that equivalent standards are met for SAPR where SARCs are not installation-based but instead work within operational and/or deployable organizations.

d. Establish guidance to meet the SAPR training requirements for legal, military criminal investigative organization (MCIO), DoD law enforcement, responders, and other Service members in Enclosure 10 of this Instruction.

e. Upon request, submit a copy of SAPR training programs or SAPR training elements to the USD(P&R) through SAPRO for evaluation of consistency and compliance with DoD SAPR training standards in this Instruction. The Military Departments will correct USD(P&R) identified DoD SAPR policy and training standards discrepancies.

f. Establish and publicize policies and procedures for reporting a sexual assault.

    (1) Require first responders (see Glossary) to be identified upon their assignment and trained, and require that their response times be continually monitored by their commanders to ensure timely response to reports of sexual assault.

    (2) Ensure established response time is based on local conditions but reflects that sexual assault victims shall be treated as emergency cases. (See Enclosure 10 of this Instruction for training requirements.)

g. Establish policy that ensures commanders are accountable for implementing and executing the SAPR program at their installations consistent with this Instruction, Reference (b), and their Service regulations.

h. Establish standards and periodic training for healthcare personnel and healthcare providers regarding the Unrestricted and Restricted Reporting options of sexual assault in accordance with Enclosure 10 of this Instruction. Enforce eligibility standards of licensed healthcare providers to perform SAFEs.

i. Establish guidance to direct that all Unrestricted Reports of violations (to include attempts) of sexual assault and non–consensual sodomy, as defined in Reference (d), against adults are immediately reported to the MCIO, regardless of the severity of the potential punishment authorized by the UCMJ.

(1) Commander(s) of the Service member(s) who is a subject of a sexual assault allegation shall provide in writing all disposition data, to include any administrative or judicial action taken, stemming from the sexual assault investigation to the MCIO.

(2) Once the investigation is completed, MCIOs shall submit case disposition data that satisfies the reporting requirements for DSAID identified in Enclosure 11 and the annual reporting requirements in Enclosure 12 of this Instruction. MCIOs shall submit case disposition data even when the sexual assault case is referred to other DoD law enforcement.

(3) A unit commander who receives an Unrestricted Report of an incident of sexual assault shall immediately refer the matter to the appropriate MCIO. A unit commander shall not conduct internal command directed investigations on sexual assault (i.e., no referrals to appointed command investigators or inquiry officers) or delay immediately contacting the MCIOs while attempting to assess the credibility of the report.

j. Establish SAPR policy that encourages commanders to be responsive to a victim's desire to discuss his or her case with the installation commander tasked by the Military Service with oversight responsibility for the SAPR program in accordance with Reference (b).

k. Establish standards for command assessment of organizational SAPR climate, including periodic follow-up assessments. Adhere to USD(P&R) SAPR guidance and effectiveness of SAPR training, awareness, prevention, and response policies and programs.

l. As a shared responsibility with ASD(HA), direct installation commanders to maintain an adequate supply of SAFE Kits in all locations where SAFEs are conducted, including deployed locations. Direct that Military Service SAPR personnel, to include medical personnel, are appropriately trained on protocols for the use of the SAFE Kit and comply with prescribed chain of custody procedures described in their Military Service-specific MCIO procedures.

m. Establish procedures that require, upon seeking assistance from a SARC, SAPR VA, MCIO, the Victim Witness Assistance Program (VWAP), or trial counsel, that each Service member who reports that he or she has been a victim of a sexual assault be informed of and given the opportunity to:

(1) Consult with legal assistance counsel, and in cases where the victim may have been involved in collateral misconduct (see Glossary), to consult with defense counsel.

    (a) When the alleged perpetrator is the commander or in the victim's chain of command, such victims shall be informed of the opportunity to go outside the chain of command to report the offense to other commanding officers or an Inspector General. Victims shall be informed that they can also seek assistance from the DoD Safe Helpline (see Glossary).

    (b) The victim shall be informed that legal assistance is optional and may be declined, in whole or in part, at any time.

    (c) Commanders shall require that information and services concerning the investigation and prosecution be provided to victims in accordance with VWAP procedures in DoDI 1030.2 (Reference (x)).

(2) Have a SARC or SAPR VA present when law enforcement or defense counsel interviews the victim.

n. Establish procedures to ensure that, in the case of a general or special court-martial involving a sexual assault as defined in Reference (b), a copy of the prepared record of the proceedings of the court-martial (not to include sealed materials, unless otherwise approved by the presiding military judge or appellate court) shall be given to the victim of the offense if the victim testified during the proceedings. The record of the proceedings (prepared in accordance with Service regulations) shall be provided without charge and as soon as the record is authenticated. The victim shall be notified of the opportunity to receive the record of the proceedings in accordance with Reference (l).

o. The commanders shall also require that a completed DD Form 2701, "Initial Information for Victims and Witnesses of Crime," be distributed to the victim by DoD law enforcement agents. (DD Form 2701 may be obtained via the Internet at http://www.dtic.mil/whs/directives/infomgt/forms/eforms/dd2701.pdf.)

p. Establish procedures to require commanders to protect the SARC and SAPR VA from coercion, retaliation, and reprisals, related to the execution of their duties and responsibilities.

q. Establish procedures to protect victims of sexual assault from coercion, retaliation, and reprisal in accordance with DoDD 7050.06 (Reference (y)).

r. Establish Military Service-specific guidance to ensure collateral misconduct is addressed in a manner that is consistent and appropriate to the circumstances, and at a time that encourages continued victim cooperation.

s. Establish expedited transfer procedures for victims of sexual assault in accordance with paragraph 4.r. above the signature of this Instruction and Enclosure 5 of this Instruction.

t. Appoint a representative to the SAPR integrated product team (IPT) in accordance with Enclosure 3 of this Instruction, and provide chairs or co-chairs for working integrated product teams (WIPT), when requested. Appoint a representative to SAPRO oversight teams upon request.

u. Provide quarterly and annual reports of sexual assault involving Service members to Director, SAPRO, to be consolidated into the annual Secretary of Defense report to Congress in accordance with Reference (b) and sections 113 and 4331 of Reference (d). (See Enclosure 12 of this Instruction for reporting requirements.)

v. Provide budget program and obligation data, as requested by the DoD SAPRO.

w. Require that reports of sexual assault be entered into DSAID through interface with a Military Service data system or by direct data entry by SARCs.

   (1) Data systems that interface with DSAID shall be modified and maintained to accurately provide information to DSAID.

   (2) Only SARCs who have, at a minimum, a favorable NAC shall be permitted access to enter sexual assault reports into DSAID.

x. Provide Director, SAPRO, a written description of any sexual assault related research projects contemporaneous with commencing the actual research. When requested, provide periodic updates on results and insights. Upon conclusion of such research, a summary of the findings will be provided to DoD SAPRO as soon as practicable.

y. Establish procedures for supporting the DoD Safe Helpline in accordance with each Military Service-specific MOU or MOA between SAPRO and the Military Departments, to include but not limited to, providing and updating SARC contact information for the referral DoD Safe Helpline database; providing timely response to victim feedback; and publicizing the DoD Safe Helpline to SARCs and Service members.

   (1) Utilize the DoD Safe Helpline as the sole DoD hotline to provide crisis intervention, facilitate victim reporting through connection to the nearest SARC, and other resources as warranted.

   (2) The DoD Safe Helpline does not replace local base and installation SARC or SAPR VA contact information.

z. Establish procedures to implement SAPR training in accordance with Enclosure 10 of this Instruction, to include prevention and response.

aa. Require that reports of sexual assaults are provided to the Commanders of the Combatant Commands for their respective area of responsibility on a quarterly basis, or as requested.

ab. For CMGs:

(1) Require the installation commander or the deputy installation commander chair the multi-disciplinary CMG (see Enclosure 9 of this Instruction) on a monthly basis to review individual cases of Unrestricted Reporting of sexual assault, facilitate monthly victim updates, direct system coordination, accountability, and victim access to quality services. This responsibility may not be delegated.

(2) Require that the installation SARC (in the case of multiple SARCs on an installation, then the Lead SARC) serve as the co-chair of the CMG. This responsibility may not be delegated.

(3) If the installation is a joint base or if the installation has tenant commands, the commander of the tenant organization and their designated Lead SARC shall be invited to the CMG meetings. The commander of the tenant organization shall provide appropriate information to the host commander, to enable the host commander to provide the necessary supporting services.

(4) The Secretaries of the Military Departments shall issue guidance to ensure that equivalent standards are met for case oversight by CMGs in situations where SARCs are not installation-based but instead work within operational and/or deployable organizations.

ac. Establish document retention procedures for Unrestricted and Restricted Reports of sexual assault in accordance with paragraph 4.p. above the signature of this Instruction.

ad. When drafting MOUs or MOAs with local civilian medical facilities to provide DoD-reimbursable healthcare (to include psychological care) and forensic examinations for Service members and TRICARE eligible sexual assault victims, require commanders to include the following provisions:

(1) Ask the victim whether he or she would like the SARC to be notified, and if yes, a SARC or SAPR VA shall respond.

(2) Local private or public sector providers shall have processes and procedures in place to assess that local community standards meet

or exceed those set forth in Reference (w) as a condition of the MOUs or MOAs.

ae. Comply with collective bargaining obligations, if applicable.

af. Provide SAPR training and education for civilian employees of the military departments in accordance with Section 585 of Reference (l).

7. CHIEF, NATIONAL GUARD BUREAU (NGB). The Chief, NGB, shall on behalf of the Secretaries of the Army and Air Force, in coordination with DoD SAPRO and the State Adjutants General, establish and implement SAPR policy and procedures for NG members on duty pursuant to title 32, United States Code (Reference (z)).

8. CHAIRMAN OF THE JOINT CHIEFS OF STAFF. The Chairman of the Joint Chiefs of Staff shall monitor implementation of this Instruction and Reference (b).

9. COMMANDERS OF THE COMBATANT COMMANDS. The Commanders of the Combatant Commands, through the Chairman of the Joint Chiefs of Staff and in coordination with the other Heads of the DoD Components, shall:

a. Require that a SAPR capability provided by the Executive Agent (see Glossary) is incorporated into operational planning guidance in accordance with Reference (b) and this Instruction.

b. Require the establishment of an MOU, MOA, or equivalent support agreement with the Executive Agent in accordance with Reference (b) and this Instruction and requires at a minimum:

(1) Coordinated efforts and resources, regardless of the location of the sexual assault, to direct optimal and safe administration of Unrestricted and Restricted Reporting options with appropriate protection, medical care, counseling, and advocacy.

(a) Ensure a 24 hour per day, 7 day per week response capability. Require first responders to respond in a timely manner.

(b) Response times shall be based on local conditions; however, sexual assault victims shall be treated as emergency cases.

(2) Notice to the SARC of every incident of sexual assault on the military installation, so that a SARC or SAPR VA can respond and offer the victim SAPR services. In situations where a sexual assault victim receives medical care and a SAFE outside of a military installation

through a MOU or MOA with a local private or public sector entities, as part of the MOU or MOA, victims shall be asked whether they would like the SARC to be notified, and if yes, the SARC or SAPR VA shall be notified and shall respond.

Oversight of the SAPR Program

(1) DIRECTOR, SAPRO. The Director, SAPRO, under the authority, direction and control of the USD(P&R) through the Director, DoDHRA, shall serve as the single point of authority, accountability, and oversight for the DoD SAPR program. DoD SAPRO provides recommendations to the USD(P&R) on the issue of DoD sexual assault policy matters on prevention, response, oversight, standards, training, and program requirements. The Director, SAPRO, shall:

   a. Assist the USD(P&R) in developing, administering, and monitoring the effectiveness of DoD SAPR policies and programs. Implement and monitor compliance with DoD sexual assault policy on prevention and response.

   b. With the USD(P&R), update the Deputy Secretary of Defense on SAPR policies and programs on a semi-annual schedule.

   c. Develop DoD programs to direct SAPR education, training, and awareness for DoD personnel consistent with this Instruction and Reference (b).

   d. Coordinate the management of DoD SAPR Program and oversee the implementation in the Service SAPR Programs.

   e. Provide technical assistance to the Heads of the DoD Components in addressing matters concerning SAPR and facilitate the identification and resolution of issues and concerns common to the Military Services and joint commands.

   f. Develop strategic program guidance, joint planning objectives, standard terminology, and identify legislative changes needed to advance the SAPR program.

   g. Develop oversight metrics to measure compliance and effectiveness of SAPR training, sexual assault awareness, prevention, and response policies and programs; analyze data; and make recommendations regarding SAPR policies and programs to the USD(P&R) and the Secretaries of the Military Departments.

   h. Establish reporting categories and monitor specific goals included in the annual SAPR assessments of each Military Service and its respective Military Service Academy, as required by Reference (b), sections 113 and 4331 of Reference (d), and in accordance with Enclosure 12 of this Instruction.

i. Acquire quarterly, annual, and installation-based SAPR data from the Military Services and assemble annual congressional reports involving persons covered by this Instruction and Reference (b). Consult with and rely on the Secretaries of the Military Departments in questions concerning disposition results of sexual assault cases in their respective Military Departments.

j. Prepare the annual fiscal year (FY) reports submitted by the Secretary of Defense to the Congress on the sexual assaults involving Service members and a report on the members of the Military Service Academies to Congress submitted by the Secretary of Defense.

k. Publicize SAPR outreach, awareness, prevention, response, and oversight initiatives and programs.

l. Oversee the development, implementation, maintenance, and function of the DSAID to meet congressional reporting requirements, support Military Service SAPR program management, and conduct DoD SAPRO oversight activities.

m. Establish, oversee, publicize, and maintain the DoD Safe Helpline and facilitate victim reporting through its connection to the nearest SARC, and other resources as warranted.

n. Establish and oversee the D-SAACP to ensure all sexual assault victims are offered the assistance of a credentialed SARC or SAPR VA.

o. Annually review the Military Services resourcing and funding of the U.S. Army Criminal Investigation Laboratory (USACIL) in the area of sexual assault.

  (1) Assist the Department of the Army in identifying the funding and resources needed to operate USACIL, to facilitate forensic evidence being processed within 60 working days from day of receipt in accordance with section 113 of Reference (d).

  (2) Encourage the Military Services that use USACIL to contribute to the operation of USACIL by ensuring that USACIL is funded and resourced appropriately to complete forensic evidence processing within 60 working days.

p. Chair the SAPR IPT.

2. SAPR IPT

a. Membership. The SAPR IPT shall include:
  (1) Director, SAPRO. The Director shall serve as the chair.
  (2) Deputy Assistant Secretaries for Manpower and Reserve Affairs of the Departments of the Army and the Air Force.
  (3) A senior representative of the Department of the Navy SAPRO.
  (4) A G/FO or DoD SES civilian from: the Joint Staff, Manpower and Personnel (J-1); the Office of the Assistant Secretary of Defense for Reserve Affairs; the NGB; the Office of the General Counsel, DoD; and the Office of the Assistant Secretary of Defense for Health Affairs.
      Other DoD Components representatives shall be invited to specific SAPR IPT meetings when their expertise is needed to inform and resolve issues being addressed. A senior representative from the Coast Guard shall be an invited guest.
  (5) Consistent with Section 8(c) of title 5, U.S.C. (also known as the "Inspector General Act of 1978") (Reference (aa)), the IG DoD shall be authorized to send one or more observers to attend all SAPR IPT meetings in order to monitor and evaluate program performance.

b. Duties. The SAPR IPT shall:
  (1) Through the chair, advise the USD(P&R) and the Secretary of Defense on SAPR IPT meeting recommendations on policies for sexual assault issues involving persons covered by this Instruction.
  (2) Serve as the implementation and oversight arm of the DoD SAPR Program. Coordinate policy and review the DoD's SAPR policies and programs consistent with this Instruction and Reference (b), as necessary. Monitor the progress of program elements.
  (3) Meet every other month. Ad hoc meetings may be scheduled as necessary at the discretion of the chair. Members are selected and meetings scheduled according to the SAPR IPT Charter.
  (4) Discuss and analyze broad SAPR issues that may generate targeted topics for WIPTs. WIPTs shall focus on one select issue, be governed by a charter with enumerated goals for which the details will be laid out in individual work plans (see Glossary), and be subject to a definitive timeline for the accomplishment of the stated goals. Issues that cannot be resolved by the SAPR IPT or that require higher level decision making shall be sent to the USD(P&R) for resolution.

c. Chair Duties. The chair shall:

    (1) Advise the USD(P&R) and the Secretary of Defense on SAPR IPT recommendations on policies for sexual assault issues involving persons covered by this Instruction.

    (2) Represent the USD(P&R) in SAPR matters consistent with this Instruction and Reference (b).

    (3) Oversee discussions in the SAPR IPT that generate topics for WIPTs. Provide final approval for topics, charters, and timelines for WIPTs.

Chain of command

Unrestricted Reports to Commanders. The SARC shall provide the installation commander of sexual assault victims with information regarding all Unrestricted Reports within 24 hours of an Unrestricted Report of sexual assault. This notification may be extended by the commander to 48 hours after the Unrestricted Report of the incident when there are extenuating circumstances in deployed environments.

Restricted Reports to Commanders. For the purposes of public safety and command responsibility, in the event of a Restricted Report, the SARC shall report non-PII concerning sexual assault incidents (without information that could reasonably lead to personal identification of the victim or the alleged assailant (see exception of subparagraph 5.b.(2) of this enclosure) only to the installation commander within 24 hours of the report. This notification may be extended by the commander to 48 hours after the Restricted Report of the incident when there are extenuating circumstances in deployed environments. The SARC's communications with victims are protected by the Restricted Reporting option and the MRE 514, established in Executive Order 13593 (Reference (ac)).

    (1) Even if the victim chooses not to pursue an investigation, Restricted Reporting gives the installation commander a clearer picture of the reported sexual assaults within the command. The installation commander can then use the information to enhance preventive measures, to enhance the education and training of the command's personnel, and to scrutinize more closely the organization's climate and culture for contributing factors.

    (2) Neither the installation commander nor DoD law enforcement may use the information from a Restricted Report for investigative purposes or in a manner that is likely to discover, disclose, or reveal the identities of the victims unless an exception applies.

Improper disclosure of Restricted Reporting information may result in discipline pursuant to the UCMJ or other adverse personnel or administrative actions.

EXCEPTIONS TO RESTRICTED REPORTING AND DISCLOSURES

The SARC will evaluate the confidential information provided under the Restricted Report to determine whether an exception applies.

(1) The SARC shall disclose the otherwise protected confidential information only after consultation with the staff judge advocate (SJA) of the installation commander, supporting judge advocate or other legal advisor concerned, who shall advise the SARC whether an exception to Restricted Reporting applies. In addition, the SJA, supporting judge advocate, or other legal advisor concerned will analyze the impact of MRE 514 on the communications.

(2) When there is uncertainty or disagreement on whether an exception to Restricted Reporting applies, the matter shall be brought to the attention of the installation commander for decision without identifying the victim (using non-PII information). Improper disclosure of confidential communications under Restricted Reporting, improper release of medical information, and other violations of this guidance are prohibited and may result in discipline pursuant to the UCMJ or State statute, loss of privileges, loss of certification or credentialing, or other adverse personnel or administrative actions.

The following exceptions to the prohibition against disclosures of Restricted Reporting authorize a disclosure of a Restricted Report only if one or more of the following conditions apply:

(1) Authorized by the victim in writing.

(2) Necessary to prevent or mitigate a serious and imminent threat to the health or safety of the victim or another person; for example, multiple reports involving the same alleged suspect (repeat offender) could meet this criteria. See similar safety and security exceptions in MRE 514 (Reference (ac)).

(3) Required for fitness for duty or disability determinations. This disclosure is limited to only the information necessary to process duty or disability determinations for Service members.

(4) Required for the supervision of coordination of direct victim treatment or services. The SARC, SAPR VA, or healthcare personnel can disclose specifically requested information to those

individuals with an official need to know, or as required by law or regulation.

Ordered by a military official (e.g., a duly authorized trial counsel subpoena in a UCMJ case), Federal or State judge, or as required by a Federal or State statute or applicable U.S. international agreement. The SARC, SAPR VA, and healthcare personnel will consult with privileged information, to determine if the exception criteria apply and whether a duty to disclose the otherwise protected information is present. Until those determinations are made, only non-PII shall be disclosed.

Healthcare personnel may also convey to the victim's unit commander any possible adverse duty impact related to the victim's medical condition and prognosis in accordance with DoD Directive 5400.11 (Reference (ad)). However, such circumstances do NOT otherwise warrant a Restricted Reporting exception to policy. Therefore, the confidential communication related to the sexual assault may not be disclosed. Improper disclosure of confidential communications, improper release of medical information, and other violations of this Instruction and Reference (b) are prohibited and may result in discipline pursuant to the UCMJ or State statute, loss of privileges, or other adverse personnel or administrative actions.

The SARC or SAPR VA shall inform the victim when a disclosure in accordance with the exceptions in this section of this enclosure is made.

If a SARC, SAPR VA, or healthcare personnel make an unauthorized disclosure of a confidential communication, that person is subject to disciplinary action. Unauthorized disclosure has no impact on the status of the Restricted Report. All Restricted Reporting information is still confidential and protected. However, unauthorized or inadvertent disclosures made to a commander or law enforcement shall result in notification to the MCIO.

ACTIONABLE RIGHTS. Restricted Reporting does not create any actionable rights for the victim or alleged offender or constitute a grant of immunity for any actionable conduct by the offender or the victim.

Commander and Management SAPR Procedures

SAPR MANAGEMENT. Commanders, supervisors, and managers at all levels are responsible for the effective implementation of the SAPR program and policy. Military and DoD civilian officials at each management level shall advocate a strong SAPR program and provide education and training that shall enable them to prevent and appropriately respond to incidents of sexual assault.

INSTALLATION COMMANDER SAPR RESPONSE PROCEDURES. Each installation commander shall develop guidelines to establish a 24 hour, 7 day per week sexual assault response capability for their locations, including deployed areas. For SARCs that operate within deployable commands that are not attached to an installation, senior commanders of the deployable commands shall ensure that equivalent SAPR standards are met.

COMMANDER SAPR RESPONSE PROCEDURES. Each Commander shall:

a. Encourage the use of the commander's sexual assault response protocols for Unrestricted Reports as the baseline for commander's response to the victim, an offender, and proper response of a sexual assault within a unit. The Commander's Sexual Assault Response Protocols for Unrestricted Reports of Sexual Assault are located in the SAPR Policy Toolkit, on www.sapr.mil. These protocols may be expanded to meet Military Service-specific requirements and procedures.

b. Meet with the SARC within 30 days of taking command for one-on-one SAPR training. The training shall include a trends brief for unit and area of responsibility and the confidentiality requirements in Restricted Reporting. The commander must contact the judge advocate for training on the MRE 514 privilege.

c. Require the SARC to:

(1) Be notified of every incident of sexual assault involving Service members or persons covered in this Instruction, in or outside of the military installation when reported to DoD personnel. When notified, the SARC or SAPR VA shall respond to offer the victim SAPR services. All SARCs shall be authorized to perform victim advocate duties in accordance with service regulations, and will be acting in the performance of those duties.

(a) In Restricted Reports, the SARC shall be notified by the healthcare personnel or the SAPR VA.

(b) In Unrestricted Reports, the SARC shall be notified by the DoD responders.

(2) Provide the installation commander with information regarding an Unrestricted Report within 24 hours of an Unrestricted Report of sexual assault.

(3) Provide the installation commander with non-PII, as defined in the Glossary, within 24 hours of a Restricted Report of sexual assault. This notification may be extended to 48 hours after the report of the incident if there are extenuating circumstances in the

deployed environment. Command and installation demographics shall be taken into account when determining the information to be provided.

(4) Be supervised and evaluated by the installation commander or deputy installation commander in the performance of SAPR procedures in accordance with Enclosure 6 of this Instruction.

(5) Receive SARC training to follow procedures in accordance with Enclosure 6 of this Instruction. Upon implementation of the D–SAACP, standardized criteria for the selection and training of SARCs and SAPR VAs shall comply with specific Military Service guidelines and certification requirements, when implemented by SAPRO.

(6) Follow established procedures to store the DD Form 2910 pursuant to Military Service regulations regarding the storage of documents with PII. (Copies may be obtained via the Internet at http://www.dtic.mil/whs/directives/infomgt/forms/eforms/dd2910.pdf.) Follow established procedures to store the original DD Form 2910 and ensure that all Federal and Service privacy regulations are adhered to.

d. Evaluate medical personnel per Military Service regulation in the performance of SAPR procedures as described in Enclosure 7 of this Instruction.

e. Require adequate supplies of SAFE Kits be maintained by the active component. The supplies shall be routinely evaluated to guarantee adequate numbers to meet the need of sexual assault victims.

f. Require DoD law enforcement and healthcare personnel to comply with prescribed chain of custody procedures described in their Military Service-specific MCIO procedures. Modified procedures applicable in cases of Restricted Reports of sexual assault are explained in Enclosure 8 of this Instruction.

g. Require that a CMG is conducted on a monthly basis in accordance with Enclosure 9 of this Instruction.

(1) Chair or attend the CMG, as appropriate. Direct the required CMG members to attend.

(2) Commanders shall provide victims of a sexual assault who filed an Unrestricted Report monthly updates regarding the current status of any ongoing investigative, medical, legal, or command proceedings regarding the sexual assault until the final disposition of the reported assault, and to the extent permitted pursuant to

Reference (x), Public Law 104-191, and section 552a of title 5, U.S.C. (References (ae) and (af)). This is a non–delegable commander duty. This update must occur within 72 hours of the last CMG. Commanders of the NG victims who were sexually assaulted when the victim was on title 10 orders and filed unrestricted reports are required to update, to the extent allowed by law and regulations, the victim's home State title 32 commander as to all or any ongoing investigative, medical, and legal proceedings regarding the extent of any actions being taken by the active component against subjects who remain on title 10 orders.

h. Ensure that resolution of Unrestricted Report sexual assault cases shall be expedited.

(1) A unit commander who receives an Unrestricted Report of a sexual assault shall immediately refer the matter to the appropriate MCIO, to include any offense identified by Reference (d). A unit commander shall not conduct internal command directed investigations on sexual assault (i.e., no referrals to appointed command investigators or inquiry officers) or delay immediately contacting the MCIOs while attempting to assess the credibility of the report.

(2) The final disposition of a sexual assault shall immediately be reported by the commander to the assigned MCIO. Dispositions on cases referred by MCIOs to other DoD law enforcement agencies shall be immediately reported to the MCIOs upon their final disposition. MCIOs shall request dispositions on referred cases from civilian law enforcement agencies and, if received, those dispositions shall be immediately reported by the MCIO in DSAID in order to meet the congressional annual reporting requirements. When requested by MCIOs and other DoD law enforcement, commanders shall provide final disposition of sexual assault cases. Final case disposition is required to be inputted into DSAID.

(3) If the MCIO has been notified of the disposition in a civilian sexual assault case, the MCIO shall notify the commander of this disposition immediately.

i. Appoint a point of contact to serve as a formal liaison between the installation SARC and the installation family advocacy program (FAP) and domestic violence intervention and prevention staff (or civilian domestic resource if FAP is not available for a Reserve Component victim) to direct coordination when a sexual assault occurs within a domestic relationship or involves child abuse.

j. Ensure appropriate training of all military responders be directed and documented in accordance with training standards in Enclosure 10 of this Instruction. Direct and document appropriate training of all military responders who attend the CMG.

k. Identify and maintain a liaison with civilian sexual assault victim resources. Where necessary, it is strongly recommended that an MOU or MOAs with the appropriate local authorities and civilian service organizations be established to maximize cooperation, reciprocal reporting of sexual assault information, and consultation regarding jurisdiction for the prosecution of Service members involved in sexual assault, as appropriate.

l. Require that each Service member who reports a sexual assault, pursuant to the respective Military Service regulations, be given the opportunity to consult with legal assistance counsel, and in cases where the victim may have been involved in collateral misconduct, to consult with defense counsel. Victims shall be referred to VWAP. Information concerning the prosecution shall be provided to victims in accordance with VWAP procedures in Reference (y). The Service member victim shall be informed of this opportunity to consult with legal assistance counsel as soon as the victim seeks assistance from a SARC, SAPR VA, or any DoD law enforcement agent or judge advocate.

m. Direct that DoD law enforcement agents and VWAP personnel provide victims of sexual assault who elect an Unrestricted Report the information outlined in DoDD 1030.01 (Reference (ag)) and Reference (aa) throughout the investigative and legal process. The completed DD Form 2701 shall be distributed to the victim in Unrestricted Reporting cases by DoD law enforcement agents.

n. Require that MCIOs utilize the investigation descriptions found in the Appendix to Enclosure 12 in this Instruction.

o. Establish procedures to ensure that in the case of a general or special court-martial involving a sexual assault as defined in Reference (b), a copy of the prepared record of the proceedings of the court-martial (not to include sealed materials, unless otherwise approved by the presiding military judge or appellate court) shall be given to the victim of the offense if the victim testified during the proceedings. The record of the proceedings (prepared in accordance with Service regulations) shall be provided without charge and as soon as the record is authenticated. The victim shall be notified of the opportunity to receive the record of the proceedings in accordance with Reference (1).

p. Protect sexual assault victims from coercion, discrimination, or reprisals. Commanders shall protect SARCs and SAPR VAs from coercion, discrimination, or reprisals related to the execution of their SAPR duties and responsibilities.

q. Require that sexual assault reports be entered into DSAID through interface with a Military Service data system, or by direct data entry by authorized personnel.

r. Designate an official, usually the SARC, to generate an alpha-numeric Restricted Reporting case number (RRCN).

s. Appoint a healthcare provider, as an official duty, in each MTF to be the resident point of contact concerning SAPR policy and sexual assault care.

MOUs OR MOAs WITH LOCAL CIVILIAN AUTHORITIES. The purpose of MOUs and MOAs is to:

a. Enhance communications and the sharing of information regarding sexual assault prosecutions, as well as of the sexual assault care and forensic examinations that involve Service members and eligible TRICARE beneficiaries covered by this Instruction.

b. Collaborate with local community crisis counseling centers, as necessary, to augment or enhance their sexual assault programs.

c. Provide liaison with private or public sector sexual assault councils, as appropriate.

d. Provide information about medical and counseling services related to care for victims of sexual assault in the civilian community, when not otherwise available at the MTFs, in order that military victims may be offered the appropriate healthcare and civilian resources, where available and where covered by military healthcare benefits.

e. Where appropriate or required by MOU or MOA, facilitate training for civilian service providers about SAPR policy and the roles and responsibilities of the SARC and SAPR VA.

LINE OF DUTY (LOD) PROCEDURES

a. Members of the Reserve Components, whether they file a Restricted or Unrestricted Report, shall have access to medical treatment and counseling for injuries and illness incurred from a sexual assault inflicted upon a Service member when performing active duty service, as defined in section 101(d)(3) of Reference (d), and inactive duty training.

b. Medical entitlements remain dependent on a LOD determination as to whether or not the sexual assault incident occurred in an active duty or inactive duty training status. However, regardless of their duty status at the time that the sexual assault incident occurred, or at the time that they are seeking SAPR services (see Glossary), Reserve Component members can elect either the Restricted or Unrestricted Reporting option (see Glossary in Reference (b)) and have access to the SAPR services of a SARC and a SAPR VA.

c. The following LOD procedures shall be followed by Reserve Component commanders.

(1) LOD determinations may be made without the victim being identified to DoD law enforcement or command, solely for the purpose of enabling the victim to access medical care and psychological counseling, and without identifying injuries from sexual assault as the cause.

(2) When assessing LOD determinations for sexual assault victims, the commander of the Reserve command in each component and the directors of the Army and Air NGBs shall designate individuals within their respective organizations to process LODs for victims of sexual assault when performing active service, as defined in section 101(d)(3) of Reference (d), and inactive duty training.

(a) Designated individuals shall possess the maturity and experience to assist in a sensitive situation and, if dealing with a Restricted Report, to safeguard confidential communications. These individuals are specifically authorized to receive confidential communications as defined by the Glossary of this Instruction for the purpose of determining LOD status.

(b) The appropriate SARC will brief the designated individuals on Restricted Reporting policies, exceptions to Restricted Reporting, and the limitations of disclosure of confidential communications as specified in section 5 of Enclosure 4 of this Instruction. The SARC and these individuals may consult with their servicing legal office, in the same manner as other recipients of privileged information for assistance, exercising due care to protect confidential communications by disclosing only non-identifying information. Unauthorized disclosure may result in disciplinary action, in accordance with paragraphs 4.a. and 4.b. of Enclosure 4 of this Instruction.

(3) For LOD purposes, the victim's SARC may provide documentation that substantiates the victim's duty status as well as the filing of the Restricted Report to the designated official.

(4) If medical or mental healthcare is required beyond initial treatment and follow-up, a licensed medical or mental health provider must recommend a continued treatment plan.

(5) When evaluating pay and entitlements, the modification of the LOD process for Restricted Reporting does not extend to pay and allowances or travel and transportation incident to the healthcare entitlement. However, at any time the Service member may request an unrestricted LOD to be completed in order to receive the full range of entitlements authorized pursuant to DoDI 1241.2 (Reference (ah)).

EXPEDITED VICTIM TRANSFER REQUESTS

a. Any threat to life or safety of a Service member shall be immediately reported to command and DoD law enforcement authorities (see Glossary) and a request to transfer the victim under these circumstances will be handled in accordance with established Service regulations.

b. Service members who file an Unrestricted Report of sexual assault shall be informed by the SARC, SAPR VA, or the Service member's commanding officer (CO) at the time of making the report, or as soon as practicable, of the option to request a temporary or permanent expedited transfer from their assigned command or installation, or to a different location within their assigned command or installation. The Service members shall initiate the transfer request and submit the request to their COs. The CO shall document the date and time the request is received.

(1) A presumption shall be established in favor of transferring a Service member (who initiated the transfer request) following a credible report (see Glossary) of sexual assault. The CO, or the appropriate approving authority, shall make a credible report determination at the time the expedited request is made after considering the advice of the supporting judge advocate, or other legal advisor concerned, and the available evidence based on an MCIO's investigation's information (if available).

(2) Expedited transfers of Service members who report that they are victims of sexual assault shall be limited to sexual assault offenses reported in the form of an Unrestricted Report.

(a) Sexual assault against adults is defined in the Glossary of Reference (b) and includes Article 120 and Article 125 of Reference (q). This Instruction does not address victims covered under the Family Advocacy Program in Reference (n).

(b) If the Service member files a Restricted Report in accordance with Reference (b) and requests an expedited transfer, the Service member must affirmatively change his or her reporting option to Unrestricted Reporting on the DD Form 2910, in order to be eligible for an expedited transfer.

(3) When the alleged perpetrator is the commander or otherwise in the victim's chain of command, the SARC shall inform such victims of the opportunity to go outside the chain of command to report the offense to MCIOs, other commanding officers, or an Inspector General. Victims shall be informed that they can also seek assistance from a legal assistance attorney or the DoD Safe Helpline.

(4) The CO shall expeditiously process a transfer request from a command or installation, or to a different location within the command or installation. The CO shall request and take into consideration the Service member's input before making a decision involving a temporary or permanent transfer and the location of the transfer. If approved, the transfer orders shall also include the Service member's dependents or military spouse (as applicable).

(5) The CO must approve or disapprove a Service member's request for a permanent change of station (PCS), permanent change of assignment (PCA), or unit transfer within 72 hours from receipt of the Service member's request. The decision to approve the request shall be immediately forwarded to the designated activity that processes PCS, PCA, or unit transfers (see Glossary).

(6) If the Service member's transfer request is disapproved by the CO, the Service member shall be given the opportunity to request review by the first G/FO in the chain of command of the member, or an SES equivalent (if applicable). The decision to approve or disapprove the request for transfer must be made within 72 hours of submission of the request for review. If a civilian SES equivalent reviewer approves the transfer, the Secretary of the Military Department concerned shall process and issue orders for the transfer.

(7) Military Departments shall make every reasonable effort to minimize disruption to the normal career progression of a Service member who reports that he or she is a victim of a sexual assault.

(8) Expedited transfer procedures require that a CO or the appropriate approving authority make a determination and provide his or her reasons and justification on the transfer of a Service member based on a credible report of sexual assault. A CO shall consider:

(a) The Service member's reasons for the request.

(b) Potential transfer of the alleged offender instead of the Service member requesting the transfer.

(c) Nature and circumstances of the offense.

(d) Whether a temporary transfer would meet the Service member's needs and the operational needs of the unit.

(e) Training status of the Service member requesting the transfer.

(f) Availability of positions within other units on the installation.

(g) Status of the investigation and potential impact on the investigation and future disposition of the offense, after consultation with the investigating MCIOs.

(h) Location of the alleged offender.

(i) Alleged offender's status (Service member or civilian).

(j) Other pertinent circumstances or facts.

(9) Service members requesting the transfer shall be informed that they may have to return for the prosecution of the case, if the determination is made that prosecution is the appropriate command action.

(10) Commanders shall directly counsel the Service member to ensure that he or she is fully informed regarding:

(a) Reasonably foreseeable career impacts.

(b) The potential impact of the transfer or reassignment on the investigation and case disposition or the initiation of other adverse action against the alleged offender.

(c) The effect on bonus recoupment (if, for example, they cannot work in their Air Force Specialty or Military Occupational Specialty).

(d) Other possible consequences of granting the request.

(11) Require that expedited transfer procedures for Reserve Component, Army NG, and Air NG members who make Unrestricted Reports of sexual assault be established within available resources and authorities. If requested by the Service member, the command should allow for separate training on different weekends or times from the alleged offender or with a different unit in the home drilling location to ensure undue burden is not placed on the Service

member and his or her family by the transfer. Potential transfer of the alleged offender instead of the Service member should also be considered. At a minimum, the alleged offender's access to the Service member who made the Unrestricted Report shall be controlled, as appropriate.

(12) Even in those court-martial cases in which the accused has been acquitted, the standard for approving an expedited transfer still remains whether a credible report has been filed. The commander shall consider all the facts and circumstances surrounding the case and the basis for the transfer request.

MILITARY PROTECTIVE ORDERS (MPO). In Unrestricted Reporting cases, commanders shall execute the following procedures regarding MPOs:

    a. Require the SARC or the SAPR VA to inform sexual assault victims protected by an MPO, in a timely manner, of the option to request transfer from the assigned command in accordance with section 567(c) of Reference (j).

    b. Notify the appropriate civilian authorities of the issuance of an MPO and of the individuals involved in the order, in the event an MPO has been issued against a Service member and any individual involved in the MPO does not reside on a military installation at any time during the duration of the MPO pursuant to Reference (i).

(1) An MPO issued by a military commander shall remain in effect until such time as the commander terminates the order or issues a replacement order.

(2) The issuing commander shall notify the appropriate civilian authorities of any change made in a protective order, or its termination, covered by chapter 80 of Reference (d) and the termination of the protective order.

(3) When an MPO has been issued against a Service member and any individual involved in the MPO does not reside on a military installation at any time during the duration of the MPO, notify the appropriate civilian authorities of the issuance of an MPO and of the individuals involved in the order. The appropriate civilian authorities shall include, at a minimum, the local civilian law enforcement agency or agencies with jurisdiction to respond to an emergency call from the residence of any individual involved in the order.

   c. Advise the person seeking the MPO that the MPO is not enforceable by civilian authorities off base and that victims desiring protection off base should seek a civilian protective order (CPO). Off base violations of the MPO should be reported to the issuing commander, DoD law enforcement, and the relevant MCIO for investigation.

      (1) Pursuant to section 1561a of Public Law 107-311 (Reference (ai)), a CPO shall have the same force and effect on a military installation as such order has within the jurisdiction of the court that issued such order. Commanders, MCIOs, and installation DoD law enforcement personnel shall take all reasonable measures necessary to ensure that a CPO is given full force and effect on all DoD installations within the jurisdiction of the court that issued such order.

      (2) If the victim has informed the SARC of an existing CPO, a commander shall require the SARC to inform the CMG of the existence of the CPO and its requirements. After the CPO information is received at the CMG, DoD law enforcement agents shall be required to document CPOs for all Service members in their investigative case file, to include documentation for Reserve Component personnel in title 10 status.

   d. Note that MPOs in cases other than sexual assault matters may have separate requirements.

   e. Issuing commanders fill out the DD Form 2873, "Military Protective Order (MPO)," and provide victims and alleged offenders with copies of the completed form. Verbal MPOs can be issued, but need to be subsequently documented with a DD Form 2873, as soon as possible.

   f. Require DoD law enforcement agents document MPOs for all Service members in their investigative case file, to include documentation for Reserve Component personnel in title 10 status. The appropriate DoD law enforcement agent representative to the CMG shall brief the CMG chair and co-chair on the existence of an MPO.

   g. If the commander's decision is to deny the MPO request, document the reasons for the denial. Denials of MPO requests go to the installation commander or equivalent command level (in consultation with a judge advocate) for the final decision.

COLLATERAL MISCONDUCT IN SEXUAL ASSAULT CASES

   a. Collateral misconduct by the victim of a sexual assault is one of the most significant barriers to reporting assault because of the victim's fear of punishment. Some reported sexual assaults involve circumstances where the victim may have engaged in some form of misconduct (e.g., underage drinking or other related alcohol offenses, adultery, fraternization, or other violations of certain regulations or orders). Commanders shall have discretion to defer action on alleged collateral misconduct by the sexual assault victim (and shall not be penalized for such a deferral decision), until final disposition of the sexual assault case, taking into account the trauma to the victim and responding appropriately so as to encourage reporting of sexual assault and continued victim cooperation, while also bearing in mind any potential speedy trial and statute of limitations concerns.

b. In accordance with Secretary of Defense Memorandum (Reference [aj]), the initial disposition authority is withheld from all commanders within the Department of Defense who do not possess at least special court-martial convening authority and who are not in the grade of 0-6 (i.e., colonel or Navy captain) or higher, with respect to the alleged offenses of rape, sexual assault, forcible sodomy, and all attempts to commit such offenses, in violation of Articles 120, 125, and 80 of Reference (q). Commanders may defer taking action on a victim's alleged collateral misconduct arising from or that relates to the sexual assault incident until the initial disposition action for the sexual assault investigation is completed.

c. Commanders and supervisors should take appropriate action for the victim's alleged collateral misconduct (if warranted), responding appropriately in order to encourage sexual assault reporting and continued cooperation, while avoiding those actions that may further traumatize the victim. Ultimately, victim cooperation should significantly enhance timely and effective investigations, as well as the appropriate disposition of sexual assaults.

d. Subordinate commanders shall be advised that taking action on a victim's alleged collateral misconduct may be deferred until final disposition of the sexual assault case. The Military Departments shall establish procedures so that commanders and supervisors are not penalized for deferring alleged collateral misconduct actions for the sexual assault victim until final disposition of the sexual assault case.

e. Commanders shall have the authority to determine, in a timely manner, how to best manage the disposition of alleged misconduct, to include making the decision to defer disciplinary actions regarding a victim's alleged collateral misconduct until after the final disposition of the sexual assault case, where appropriate. For those sexual assault cases for which the victim's alleged collateral misconduct is deferred, Military Service reporting and processing requirements should take such deferrals into consideration and allow for the time deferred to be subtracted, when evaluating whether a commander took too long to resolve the collateral misconduct.

COMMANDER SAPR PREVENTION PROCEDURES. Each commander shall implement a SAPR prevention program that:
   a. Establishes a command climate of sexual assault prevention predicated on mutual respect and trust, recognizes and embraces diversity, and values the contributions of all its Service members.
   b. Emphasizes that sexual assault is a crime and violates the core values of being a professional in the Military Services and ultimately destroys unit cohesion and the trust that is essential for mission readiness and success.
   c. Emphasizes DoD and Military Service policies on sexual assault and the potential legal consequences for those who commit such crimes.
   d. Monitors the organization's SAPR climate and responds with appropriate action toward any negative trends that may emerge.
   e. Identifies and remedies environmental factors specific to the location that may facilitate the commission of sexual assaults (e.g., insufficient lighting).
   f. Emphasizes sexual assault prevention training for all assigned personnel.
   g. Establishes prevention training that focus on identifying the behavior of potential offenders.

8

INITIATIVES TO COMBAT SEXUAL ASSAULT IN THE MILITARY

The men and women of the U.S. military deserve an environment that is free from the threat of sexual assault. Service members and their families must feel secure enough to report this crime without fear of retribution, and commanders must hold offenders appropriately accountable.

Under the leadership of Secretary of Defense Leon E. Panetta and General Martin Dempsey, the Chairman of the Joint Chiefs of Staff, the Department is actively pursuing additional policy and training changes to help address this challenging issue.

New initiatives include:

Elevating disposition authority for the most serious sexual assault offenses (rape, sexual assault, forcible sodomy, and attempts to commit those offenses) so that, at a minimum, these cases are addressed by a "Special Court-Martial Convening Authority" who is an officer at the colonel (or Navy captain) level.

This will ensure that cases of sexual assault receive a high level of command attention, given the seriousness of those offenses. This will also ensure that these cases remain within the chain of command, so that our leaders retain responsibility and accountability for the problem of sexual assault.

Establishing "Special Victim's Unit" capabilities within each of the Services, to ensure that specially trained investigators, prosecutors, and victim-witness assistance personnel are available to assist with sexual assault cases.

This will provide specially trained experts in evidence collection, interviewing, and interacting with survivors of sexual assault.

Requiring that sexual assault policies be explained to all service members within 14 days of their entrance on active duty.

> This will educate our newest members right away, so that they enter the military knowing that our culture will not tolerate sexual assault, and understand what to do in the event an offense occurs.

Allowing Reserve and National Guard personnel who have been sexually assaulted while on active duty to remain in their active-duty status in order to obtain the treatment and support afforded to active-duty members.

Requiring a record of the outcome of disciplinary and administrative proceedings related to sexual assault, and requiring that copies of those records be centrally retained.

> This will allow the Department to better track our progress in combating sexual assault in the military, and will help better identify potential patterns of misconduct and systemic issues.

Requiring commanders to conduct annual organizational climate assessments.

> This will allow commanders to measure whether they are meeting the Department's goal of a culture of professionalism and respect and zero tolerance of sexual assault.

Mandating wider public dissemination of available sexual assault resources, like the DoD "Safe Helpline." The helpline is available 24 hours a day via web, phone, or text message and is operated by the nonprofit Rape, Abuse, and Incest National Network through a contractual agreement with the Department. Between its launch in April 2011 and September 2011, the Safe Helpline assisted more than 770 individuals. The helpline can be reached at 877-995-5247 or www.safehelpline.org.

Enhancing training programs for sexual assault prevention, including training for new military commanders in handling sexual assault matters.

These initiatives build on new victim-focused policies that have been implemented in the past year, these initiatives include:

Assignment of a two-star general as the director of our Sexual Assault Prevention and Response Office.

Expansion of legal assistance for military spouses and adult military dependents, so they can file confidential reports and receive the services of a victim advocate and a sexual assault response coordinator.

Expedited transfers of victims who report a sexual assault to protect them from possible harassment and remove them from proximity to the alleged perpetrator.

Extended retention of forensic examination and investigative reports.

Establishment of a sexual assault advocate credentialing and certification program.

Expansion of sexual assault support services to military spouses and adult military dependents.

Expansion of emergency care and support services to DoD civilians stationed abroad and DoD U.S. citizen contractors in combat areas.

Increased funding for investigators and judge advocates to receive additional specialized training.

Implementation of an integrated data system for tracking sexual assault reports and managing cases.

Assessment of how the department trains commanding officers and senior enlisted leaders on sexual assault prevention and response.

Institutionalize Prevention Strategies in the Military Community: The goal of this priority is to establish a military culture free of sexual assault. The Department seeks to reduce, with the goal to eliminate, the number of sexual assaults involving service members through policy and institutionalized prevention efforts that influence knowledge, skills, and behaviors. In FY12, the Military Services implemented and continued a variety of training and education programs for service members that featured bystander intervention and other prevention methods. DoD surveys indicate that the vast majority of service members are receiving prevention training, hearing key prevention concepts, and reporting an intention to take active steps to prevent sexual assault. Although measuring the overall impact of prevention efforts is difficult, the Department uses the *WGRA* to estimate the prevalence (occurrence) of unwanted sexual contact involving service members in a given year. In the *2012 WGRA*, 6.1 percent of active-duty women and 1.2 percent of active-duty men indicated they experienced some kind of USC in the 12 months prior to being surveyed. For women, this represents a statistically significant increase over the 4.4 percent USC rate measured in 2010. The change in the USC rate for men from 2010 to 2012 was not statistically significant. The increased USC rate for women and the unchanged USC rate for men this year indicate that the Department has a persistent problem and much more work to do in preventing sexual assault in the Armed Forces. To that end, DoD SAPRO began to incorporate the 2012 Joint Chiefs of Staff (JCS) *Strategic Direction to the Joint Force on Sexual Assault Prevention and Response* into an updated *DoD-Wide SAPR Strategic*

Plan. This new approach will be structured around five multidisciplinary and complementary lines of effort: Prevention, Investigation, Accountability, Victim Assistance (Advocacy), and Assessment.

Increase the Climate of Victim Confidence Associated with Reporting: The goal of this priority is to increase the number of victims who make a report of sexual assault.

The Department strives to increase sexual assault reporting by improving service members' confidence in the military justice process, creating a positive command climate, enhancing education and training about reporting options, and reducing stigma and other barriers that deter reporting. In FY12, there were 3,374 reports of sexual assault involving service members. These reports involved one or more service members as either the victim or subject (alleged perpetrator) of an investigation. The 3,374 reports involved a range of crimes prohibited by the Uniform Code of Military Justice (UCMJ), from abusive sexual contact to rape. This represents a 6 percent increase over the 3,192 reports of sexual assault received in FY11, thus providing the Department greater opportunities to provide victim care and to ensure appropriate offender accountability.

The 3,374 reports involved 2,949 service member victims. Of the 3,374 reports of sexual assault in FY12, 2,558 were Unrestricted Reports. The Military Services initially received 981 Restricted Reports. At the request of the victim, 165 reports were converted from Restricted to Unrestricted, leaving 816 reports remaining Restricted in FY12. In April 2012, the secretary of defense directed that effective June 28, 2012, in certain sexual assault cases, the initial disposition authority for disciplinary actions taken under the UCMJ be elevated to commanders in the O-6 grade (i.e., colonel or Navy captain) or higher who possess at least special court-martial convening authority, to ensure these cases are handled by seasoned, more senior commanders with advice of legal counsel.

Improve Sexual Assault Response: The goal of this priority is to improve the quality of the Department's response to victims of sexual assault through programs, policies, and activities that advance victim care and enhance victims' experience with the criminal investigative and military justice processes. In FY12, the DoD Safe Helpline, the Department's confidential 24/7 hotline resource for sexual assault victims, received more than 49,000 unique visitors to its website and more than 4,600 individuals received specialized care through its online chat, telephone helpline, and texting referral services. The Department also implemented several policy changes in FY12 via Directive-Type Memoranda (DTM) and the reissuance of DoD Directive (DoDD) 6495.01, "Sexual Assault Prevention and

Response Program." These changes included a new expedited transfer policy, providing victims who make an Unrestricted Report of sexual assault the option to request an expedited transfer from their assigned command or base. This year, 216 of 218 requests for expedited transfer were approved. Another policy change required the retention of most sexual assault records for 50 years to improve the availability of documents for service members and veterans who reported the crime. Other policy changes incorporated sexual assault victims into the definition of "emergency care" and encouraged mental healthcare referrals for victims upon first contact with medical professionals. Additionally, the Military Services began implementing the FY12 National Defense Authorization Act (NDAA) requirement to assign at least one full-time SARC and SAPR VA to each brigade or equivalent unit level. Throughout the year, the Military Services also provided updated and improved training to thousands of first responders across the Department.

Improve System Accountability: The goal of this priority is to ensure the SAPR program functions as it was intended. System accountability is achieved through data collection, analysis, and reporting of case outcomes, as well as through oversight review of SAPR program components. In FY12, the Department completed development of and deployed the Defense Sexual Assault Incident Database (DSAID), a secure, centralized, case-level data system for documenting sexual assault reports and managing cases. The Department also continued to standardize case disposition definitions, resulting in a standardized definition for the term "substantiated." At the end of FY12, the Military Services reported dispositions for 2,661 of the 3,288 military and civilian subjects receiving or waiting for a disposition for the allegations against them at the close of FY12. Investigations determined that 947 of the 2,661 subjects were either outside the legal authority of the Department or a military criminal investigative agency determined the allegations were unfounded (false or baseless).

The remaining 1,714 subjects investigated for sexual assault were presented to military commanders for consideration of disciplinary action. Of the 1,714 military subjects, commanders could not take action against 509 due to evidentiary problems. Eighty-one of the 1,714 military subjects received no disciplinary action because commanders determined the criminal allegations were unfounded (false or baseless). Commanders had sufficient evidence to take disciplinary action against 1,124 of the 1,714 military subjects. Of the 1,124 subjects, sexual assault charges were substantiated for 880 subjects for whom it was determined a sexual assault offense warranted discipline. For the remaining 244 subjects, evidence supported command action for other misconduct discovered during the sexual assault investigation (such as making a false official statement, adultery, underage drinking, or other crimes under the UCMJ), but not a sexual assault charge. Command actions for sexual assault charges and other misconduct charges included court-martial charge preferrals, nonjudicial punishment, administrative discharges, or other adverse administrative actions. Sixty-eight percent of subjects receiving disciplinary action for a sexual assault had court-martial charges preferred against them.

Improve Stakeholder Knowledge and Understanding of SAPR: The goal of this priority is to ensure stakeholders know the Department is proactively working to combat the crime of sexual assault in the military, demonstrate the Department's sustained efforts, and communicate the Department's long-term commitment to achieving its objectives. In FY12, the secretary of defense, JCS, and Military Service leadership demonstrated sustained engagement and resolve to eliminate sexual assault from the Armed Forces by promoting senior leadership involvement in SAPR programs, fostering collaboration among the Military Services and civilian stakeholders, and reinforcing ownership of both the problem and solutions. The Department reached out to victims of sexual assault, civilian advocacy groups, and veterans' organizations to inform them of SAPR program progress and gain their feedback. The secretary of defense took an active role by authoring new policies, directing the evaluation of programs, and increasing awareness of the Department's commitment to combating sexual assault.

SEXUAL ASSAULT RESPONSE COORDINATORS (SARCS) AND UNIT VICTIM COORDINATORS (UVCS)

SAPR VA SEXUAL ASSAULT RESPONSE PROTOCOLS CHECKLIST INITIAL RESPONSE

( ) Ensure that the victim understands that speaking with the VA is voluntary.
( ) Assess for imminent danger of life-threatening or physical harm to the victim by himself or herself (suicidal), by another (homicidal), or to another (homicidal).
( ) Seek immediate consultation from appropriate healthcare provider (HCP) for professional assessment when there is an imminent danger of life-threatening or physical harm to the victim or another person.

( ) If the victim has requested Restricted Reporting and the healthcare provider (HCP) determines there is an imminent danger, advise the victim of the exception to the Confidential Reporting Policy and notify the SARC.

( ) The SARC shall validate the exception and notify command and/or law enforcement as appropriate, disclosing only the details necessary to satisfy the exception.

( ) Ascertain the victim's immediate needs.

( ) Encourage the victim to seek medical consultation/examination.

( ) Ensure the victim is aware of the actions available to promote his or her safety.

( ) As appropriate, thoroughly explain to the victim each of the reporting options available to him or her, including the exceptions and/or limitations on use applicable to each.

( ) Review the DD Form 2910 if the victim is eligible to elect the Restricted Reporting option and it has been determined that none of the exceptions are applicable:

[ ] Ensure the victim acknowledges his or her understanding of the explanation of each item by initialing on the space provided by each item.

[ ] Ensure the victim indicates the reporting option that he or she elects by initialing in the space that corresponds to his or her selection. Remind the victim that failing to elect a reporting option and initial and sign the VRPS shall automatically result in an Unrestricted Report and notifications to the command and appropriate military criminal investigative organization.

[ ] If the victim elects the "Restricted Reporting option," reiterate the availability of the option to change to "Unrestricted Reporting" at any time, which will result in the notification of command and law enforcement for possible initiation of an investigation.

[ ] Advise the victim to keep a signed and dated copy of the form for the victim's records. The form may be used by the victim in other matters before other agencies or for any lawful purpose. For example, the form can be used in proceedings before the Department of Veterans Affairs to provide documentation that the victim made a Restricted Report of sexual assault even if it does not provide proof that the sexual assault actually occurred.

[ ] Ensure signature and date by the VA and the victim in the designated spaces.

[ ] Provide a copy to the victim for his or her personal safekeeping, and give the original to the SARC as soon as practicable.

( ) Offer the information, as appropriate, regarding local resources for immediate safety and long-term protection and support, workplace safety, housing, childcare, legal services, clinical resources, medical services, chaplain resources, transitional compensation, and other military and civilian support services.

( ) Facilitate victim's contact with military and civilian resources, as requested by the victim.

( ) Advise victim of availability to provide ongoing advocacy services for as long as desired.

( ) Consult with the SARC on immediate assistance provided.

ONGOING ASSISTANCE RELATED TO RECOVERY FROM SEXUAL ASSAULT

( ) Serve as a member of the case-management group and attend all Sexual Assault Case Management Group meetings involving the victim's case in order to represent the victim and to ensure the victim's needs are met.

( ) Maintain follow-up contact with the victim as requested by the victim.

( ) Support the victim in decision-making by providing relevant information and discussing available options.

( ) Assist the victim with prioritizing actions and establishing short- and long-term goals related to recovery from sexual assault.

( ) Support the victim in advocating on his or her own behalf.

( ) Provide the victim comprehensive information and referral on relevant local military and civilian resources and Safe Helpline.

( ) Assist the victim in gaining access to service providers and victim support resources that can help the victim explore future options and prioritize actions.

( ) Assist the victim in contacting appropriate military and civilian legal offices for personal legal advice and assistance specific to the victim's circumstances or case, including the filing for civilian or military protective orders. The VA shall not provide legal advice, but may provide general information on the civil or criminal legal process.

( ) Consult and work with the assigned Victim/Witness Liaison as applicable.

( ) Advise the victim of sexual assault clinical resources.

( ) Advise the victim of the impact of sexual assault on family members and offer referral information for family members.

( ) Accompany the victim to appointments and civilian and military court proceedings, as appropriate and when requested by the victim.

( ) Consult regularly with the SARC on ongoing assistance provided.

9

REDUCING YOUR
RISK OF SEXUAL ASSAULT

There are many steps you can take to help reduce your risk of being sexually assaulted. We also have some tips on how to look out for buddies and keep them safe.

ACTIVE BYSTANDER INTERVENTION

One of the most effective methods of preventing sexual assault is bystander intervention.

What Is Active Bystander Intervention?

This approach encourages people to identify situations that might lead to a sexual assault and then safely intervene to prevent an assault from occurring. Active Bystander Intervention discourages victim blaming by switching the focus of prevention to what a community of people can do collectively. The approach also allows for a change in cultural expectations by empowering everyone to say or do something when they see inappropriate or harmful behavior. This method of intervention places the responsibility of sexual assault prevention on both men and women.

How to Intervene

There are three components to Active Bystander Intervention:

Recognizing when to intervene. Some people might be concerned that they are being encouraged to place themselves in jeopardy to stop crimes in progress. This is not the case. There are many situations and events that occur prior to a sexual assault that are appropriate for intervention. Active Bystander Intervention encourages people to watch for those behaviors and situations that appear to be inappropriate, coercive, and harassing.

Considering whether the situation needs attention. The Department of Defense has chosen to link "duty" with sexual assault prevention. Service members need to understand that it is their moral duty to pay attention to situations that put their friends and coworkers at risk.

Deciding if there is a responsibility to act. A great deal of research has been done to understand the conditions that encourage people to get involved. There are situational factors that influence a person's willingness to act. These include the presence of other witnesses, the uncertainty of the situation, the apparent level of danger or risk to the victim, and the setting of the event. Personal characteristics of the bystander also contribute to a decision to act.

Help Someone You Know

When choosing what form of assistance to use, there are a variety of ways to intervene. Some of them are direct, and some of them are less obvious to the perpetrator.

Making up an excuse to get him/her out of a potentially dangerous situation

Letting a friend or coworker know that his or her actions may lead to serious consequences

Never leaving his/her side, despite the efforts of someone to get him/her alone or away from you

Using a group of friends to remind someone behaving inappropriately that his or her behavior should be respectful

Taking steps to curb someone's use of alcohol before problems occur

Calling the authorities when the situation warrants

Understanding how to safely implement the choice. Safety is paramount in Active Bystander Intervention. Usually, intervening in a group is safer than intervening individually. Also, choosing a method of intervention that de-escalates the situation is safer than attempting a confrontation. However, there is no single rule that can account for every situation. Service members must use good judgment and always put safety first.

RISK REDUCTION AND PREVENTION SAFETY

Common sense, situational awareness, and trusting your instincts will reduce your risk of being sexually assaulted. Following the tips below may decrease your chances of being attacked.

If you consume alcohol, do so in moderation.

Do not leave your beverage unattended or accept a drink from an open container.

When you are with someone, communicate clearly to ensure he or she knows your limits from the beginning. Both verbal and non-verbal (body language) communication can be used to ensure the message is understood.

If you go on a date with someone you do not know very well, tell a close friend what your plans are.

Always have extra money to get home. Have a plan for someone you can call if you need help.

If you feel uncomfortable, scared, or pressured, act quickly to end the situation. Say, "Stop it," and leave or call for help.

When you go to a party, go with a group of friends. Arrive together, watch out for each other, and leave together.

Be aware of your surroundings at all times.

Do not allow yourself to be isolated with a person you do not know or trust.

Travel with a friend or in a group.

Walk only in lighted areas after dark.

Keep the doors to homes, barracks, and cars locked.

Know where the phone is located.

You have the right to say "No" even if you:

first say "Yes," and then change your mind;

have had sex with this partner before;

have been kissing or "making out"; and

are wearing what is perceived to be "provocative" clothing.

As with any violent crime, there's nothing you can do to guarantee that you will not be a victim of sexual assault. If you are sexually assaulted, remember that it is not your fault.

There are resources available to you 24/7 through Safe Helpline. Visit the online helpline (www.safehelpline.org/online-helpline.cfm) or call 877-995-5247 (the phone number is the same inside the United States or via the Defense Switched Network [DSN]).

10

TRAINING

One way to determine if a gap exists in the military's sexual harassment "zero tolerance" policy between senior leaders and commanders who implement the policy is to review existing sexual harassment training programs and preventive tools available to future commanders.

In addition to outreach, the training of service members plays an integral role in the prevention of sexual assault. Service members received annual awareness and prevention training, per SAPR policy. Sexual assault awareness and prevention training is also a mandatory component of all accession, professional military education, and pre-command training.

FY12 witnessed criminal and other misconduct allegations reported at Lackland Air Force Base. As a result, the secretary of defense directed the Military Services to perform a comprehensive assessment of all initial military training of enlisted personnel and commissioned officers to ensure a safe and secure environment. This direction required each of the Military Services to review several key areas, including the selection, training, and oversight of basic training instructors and leaders who directly supervise initial military training. The secretary of defense also directed the Military Services to review the instructor-to-student ratio, the ratio of leaders in the chain of command to instructors, and the potential benefits of an increase in female instructors. In addition, the Military Services were directed to review their internal controls to identify and prevent inappropriate behavior throughout initial military training; student accessibility to SAPR programs; the timing, contact, and delivery of SAPR-related training; and the timing and effectiveness of processes for gathering student feedback. The Military Services reported on their findings from these assessments in the first quarter of FY13. DoD SAPRO will use the results to standardize

SAPR training core competencies and learning objectives for introductory training environments.

In FY12, the Military Services implemented a variety of prevention training and education programs for service members.

The Army continued Phase III (Achieving Cultural Change) of the "I. A.M. Strong" campaign, which focused on fostering an environment free of sexual assault and harassment. The Army revised and fielded new Sexual Harassment/Assault Response and Prevention (SHARP) training in several of the Army's professional military education curricula for enlisted soldiers and officers.

The Navy implemented Bystander Intervention Training across all applicable "A" school (technical training) locations, training 312 instructors Navy-wide, impacting 27,945 students, and delivering 1,746 sessions. Additionally, the Navy developed and executed "Take the Helm" training in 6 months for senior officers and enlisted leaders to raise SAPR program awareness, explain effective sexual assault prevention approaches, focus on leader responsibilities, and promote the command's role in creating a culture of dignity and respect.

The Marine Corps implemented a comprehensive Command Team Training program, which emphasized the responsibility of commanders to establish and maintain a positive command climate. Additionally, the Marine Corps completed "Take a Stand" training for junior noncommissioned officers (NCO) in August 2012. "Take a Stand" is a bystander intervention program that was designed to be taught by junior NCOs to young enlisted members in their units. The principles of bystander intervention were also embedded in video-based Ethical Decision Games (EDG) for required all-hands training. The EDGs are guided discussions that use fictional scenarios of sexual assault to promote candid exchanges between Marines, challenge and alter preexisting assumptions about the crime, clearly define what constitutes sexual assault, and demonstrate how sexual assault undermines the values of the Marine Corps.

The Air Force concluded its Service-wide Bystander Intervention Training, which was designed to provide airmen with knowledge to recognize potentially harmful situations and take action to mitigate possible harm to their fellow wingmen. The training concluded on June 30, 2012, and served as the Air Force and Air National Guard sexual assault awareness and prevention training for all military personnel and for civilian supervisors of military personnel. The training was designed to address three different audiences: men, women, and leaders. During each 90-minute class, instructors led participants through several scenarios to stimulate discussion about behaviors that can create environments that allow a perpetrator to act.

DOD SAFE HELPLINE

In April 2011, the Department launched the DoD Safe Helpline as a crisis support service for adult service members of the DoD community who are victims of sexual assault. The DoD Safe Helpline is available 24/7 world-wide, and users can "click, call, or text" for anonymous and confidential support. Safe Helpline is owned by the DoD and operated through a contractual agreement by the nonprofit Rape, Abuse and Incest National Network (RAINN), the nation's largest anti-sexual violence organization. Safe Helpline boasts a robust database of military, civilian, and veteran services available for referral. The database also contains SARC contact information for each Military Service, the National Guard, and the Coast Guard, as well as referral information for legal resources, chaplain support, healthcare services, DVA resources (benefit claims, health care, and National Suicide Prevention Lifeline), Military OneSource, and 1,100 civilian rape crisis affiliates. In FY12, Safe Helpline received more than 49,000 unique visitors to its website and helped more than 4,600 individuals through its online chat sessions, telephone helpline sessions, and texting referral services.

In FY12, DoD SAPRO required RAINN to incorporate a course on the neurobiology of trauma to provide Safe Helpline staff with skills to better understand and address the impact of sexual assault on a survivor's thoughts, behaviors, and relationships. Additionally, DoD SAPRO expanded the umbrella of services offered through the Safe Helpline. A mobile enhanced website was developed to respond to the growing population of mobile device users. The Department also collaborated with the DVA and the Department of Labor to connect transitioning service members (TSM) who are victims of sexual assault with resources such as counseling, assistance in benefits determinations, transitions, and employment. TSMs are defined as those service members who are within 12 months of separation or 24 months of retirement from the Armed Forces.

DoD Safe Helpline also has a Safe Helpline Mobile Application for smartphones to give members of the military community free access to resources and tools to help manage the short- and long-term effects of sexual assault. Users can also use the app to connect with live sexual assault response professionals via phone or anonymous online chat. Furthermore, the app allows users to create a customized self-care plan that, once down-loaded, may be accessed without an Internet connection.

DOD STANDARDS FOR VICTIM ASSISTANCE

In FY12, DoD SAPRO led an initiative within the Department to develop a set of broad standards to guide all DoD victim assistance-related programs. The standards, which were developed by a working group with representa-tion from 20 DoD offices, require personnel working within the military community to engage with crime and harassment victims, and use an ap-proach that emphasizes ethics, competence, and a common foundation of as-sistance services. The standards are aligned to those published by the National Victim Assistance Standards Consortium. In addition, the under secretary of defense (USD) for personnel and readiness (P&R) approved the establish-ment of a Victim Assistance Leadership Council, which will monitor the implementation of the standards and provide a forum for senior DoD leaders to exchange information and collaborate on issues affecting victims.

DoD Sexual Assault Advocate Certification Program

DoD SAPRO established and implemented the DoD Sexual Assault Advocate Certification Program (D-SAACP) in FY12. The D-SAACP is designed to standardize sexual assault response to victims and professionalize DoD victim advocacy. The program consists of three prongs:

a credentialing infrastructure for SARCs and SAPR VAs;
a framework for skill-based competencies, which identifies and orga-nizes the core knowledge, skills, and attitudes for performing sexual assault victim advocacy; and
the evaluation and oversight of SARC and SAPR VA training.

A primary objective of the D-SAACP is to ensure consistent prepa-ration of SARCs and SAPR VAs. DoD SAPRO began evaluating the Military Services' SARC and SAPR VA training in FY12, with the goal of developing standardized core competencies, learning objectives, and best practices. DoD SAPRO plans to complete its evaluation and dissemi-nate recommendations to the Military Services. Successful implementation of these components is expected to increase the consistency of training, enhance the quality of support that victims receive, and build confidence in the Department's ability to respond to sexual assault. The D-SAACP addresses a congressional mandate and is responsive to a DTF-SAMS recommendation that members of the Armed Forces who report they were sexually assaulted be afforded the assistance of a nationally certified VA.

DoD SAPRO contracted with the National Organization for Victim Assistance to aid the creation of certification standards and administer the certification process through the National Advocate Certification Program. The D-SAACP application became available to SARCs and SAPR VAs in September 2012. All SARCs and SAPR VAs must be certified by October 2013 to comply with congressional requirements; the Military Services are on track to meet this requirement.

RESPONDER TRAINING

SAPRO continues to support specialized training initiatives for responders to victims of sexual assault. For example, to improve skills in investigating and addressing sexual assault cases, the DoD provided $1.3 million in funding for a special victims unit investigations course at the U.S. Army Military Police School (USAMPS), Ft. Leonard Wood, Missouri. Attendance at this course was made available to JAs from the Military Services, the National Guard, the MCIOs, and the Coast Guard Investigative Service.

Each of the Military Services and National Guard continue first responder SAPR training. "First responders" include SARCs, SAPR VAs, commanders, legal counsel, law enforcement, and healthcare personnel. The Army trained 8,495 personnel slated for duty as a SARC or SAPR VA (including Active, Guard, and Reserve) via SHARP Mobile Training Teams using the 80-hour SHARP certification curriculum.

The Navy provided initial training to 22 new SARCs and 3,844 SAPR VAs, as well as 10 hours of refresher training to 3,020 SAPR VAs. Additionally, 4,567 active-duty SAPR VAs were trained and qualified to operate in a deployed environment.

The Marine Corps provided 38 new SARCs with the 40-hour victim advocacy training necessary for credentialing. Three hundred and seventy-two SAPR VAs and Unit VAs received victim advocacy or quarterly refresher training conducted by an installation SARC. Additionally, 84 SARCs were trained and qualified to operate in a deployed environment.

The Air Force trained 70 new SARCs in a 40-hour course, and 96 SARCs received training to operate in a deployed environment. Additionally, 5,145 SAPR VAs received training, to include deployment training.

The National Guard provided 40 hours of initial training to 79 SARCs and 799 SAPR VAs. Within the Air and Army National Guard, 170 SARCs and 38 SAPR VAs received refresher training.

Commanders

The Army provided SHARP training to 203 brigade commanders, 593 battalion commanders, and 409 command sergeants major.

Navy SARCs trained a total of 2,058 commanders on their roles and responsibilities within the Navy's SAPR program. Additionally, 296 prospective commanding and executive officers, 180 command master chiefs/chiefs of the boat, and 205 flag and general officers received SAPR training prior to assuming command or a senior leadership position.

In the Marine Corps, over 70 commanders and 50 sergeants major received SAPR training in the form of Command Team SAPR Training. Additionally, 81 general officers were trained at a SAPR General Officer Symposium, and 59 senior enlisted leaders were trained on SAPR at the Sergeants Major Symposium in FY12.

The Air Force trained 4,592 Wing, Vice Wing, and Group commanders in SAPR.

The Air National Guard trained 794 commanders in bystander intervention.

Criminal Investigators

All Military Criminal Investigation Command agents who investigate sexual assault allegations received refresher training developed by USAMPS. More than 1,600 military and civilian criminal investigators from across DoD were also trained at USAMPS on sexual assault investigative techniques.

Navy SARCs trained 264 criminal investigators on their role in the Navy SAPR program. Additionally, 95 NCIS employees, special agents, investigators, and support personnel received advanced training on sexual assault investigations.

Sixty-seven new special agents in the Marine Corps completed basic training that met DoD standards for sexual assault investigation training.

In the Air Force, 2,046 criminal investigators received Annual Periodic Sexual Assault Investigations Training, and 24 completed the Sex Crimes Investigation Training Program. Additionally, 170 criminal investigators attended the Basic Special Investigations Course, and 17 attended the Advanced General Crimes Investigation Course.

The National Guard Bureau trained 10 sexual assault investigators at the Army's Special Victims Unit Investigations course at USAMPS.

Medical Personnel

In the Army, 188 physicians, physician assistants, and registered nurses completed the Medical Command Sexual Assault Medical Forensic Examiner training.

The Department of the Navy trained 27,513 medical first responders and 132 forensic examiners for both the Navy and Marine Corps.

The Air Force provided 24,680 Air Force medics with first responder SAPR training for healthcare providers.

Judge Advocates

The Army JAG Legal Center and School provided first responder training to 757 Army JAs, including 215 Army Reserve and 135 Army National Guard JA officers. The Army also trained 454 trial counsel and 151 defense counsel in sexual assault issues.

The Naval Justice School trained 178 Navy JAs on sexual assault. Examples of courses include Prosecuting Alcohol Facilitated Sexual Assault Cases, Defending Sexual Assault Cases, and Sexual Assault Investigation and Prosecution.

The Marine Corps Trial Counsel Assistance Program trained 295 JAs in sexual assault investigation and prosecution. Most trial counsel attended at least two training sessions.

In the Air Force, the Judge Advocate General's School (TJAGS) provided formal training to over 1,400 JAs and paralegals. Additionally, over 1,000 JAGs and paralegals viewed webcasts on sexual assault–related topics, and hundreds more attended training conducted at venues other than TJAGS.

The Air National Guard trained 451 JAs in bystander intervention.

Continued Education in Recovery Care

Some victims who experience a sexual assault on active duty do not disclose until they separate or are about to separate from service. DoD SAPRO staff regularly briefed the SAPR program to incoming Wounded

Warrior Care and Transition Policy Recovery Care Coordinators and Veteran Affairs Military Sexual Trauma Coordinators. This training arrangement increases the coordinators' awareness of SAPR resources.

DoD SAPRO also continued to educate deploying mental health providers and chaplains through the Center for Deployment Psychology (CDP) at the Uniformed Services University of the Health Sciences, Bethesda, Maryland. For the past four years, CDP has invited DoD SAPRO staff to provide instruction on working with victims and the SAPR program in a deployed environment.

Sexual Assault Prior to Military Service

While the Department's primary prevention focus is to reduce the number of sexual assaults involving service members, other initiatives are underway to address special populations within the Department that may require more targeted interventions. According to long-standing civilian research, sexual victimization is a likely risk factor for subsequent victimization. Recognizing this, the Department added new items to the *2012 WGRA* to understand the extent to which service members have experienced USC *prior* to entering military service and *since* entering military service.

The *2012 WGRA* asked respondents to indicate if they had experienced USC prior to entering military service. Thirty percent of women and 6 percent of men indicated they experienced USC prior to entry into the military. Respondents were also asked to indicate if they had experienced USC since entering military service. Including experiences of USC in the past 12 months, 23 percent of women and 4 percent of men indicated they experienced USC since joining the military.

Men and women who indicated experiencing USC prior to entering the military were also overrepresented in the percentage of service members who experienced USC in the previous year. In other words, service members with a pre-service history of USC accounted for a larger-than-expected proportion of those experiencing USC.

Sexual Assault in the Military and Civilian Sectors

The Center for Disease Control (CDC) *National Intimate Partner and Sexual Violence Survey (NISVS)* is an ongoing, nationally representative telephone survey that collects detailed information on intimate partner violence (IPV), sexual violence, and stalking victimization of adult women and men in the United States. The survey collects data on both past-year and lifetime experiences of violence. The CDC developed the *NISVS* to better describe and monitor the magnitude of these forms of violence in the United States. In 2010—the initial year of the *NISVS*—the Department, Department of Justice (DOJ), and CDC worked together to include two random samples from the military: active-duty women and wives of active-duty men. Based on the survey design, the *NISVS* allowed for a first-time comparison of civilian and military rates of IPV, sexual violence, and stalking. The *NISVS* civilian sample involved about 9,000 civilian women. The *NISVS* military sample involved about 2,800 DoD women (1,408 active-duty women and 1,428 wives of active-duty men). Statistical controls were applied to ensure that age and marital differences between these three groups did not distort the survey results. The definitions of IPV, sexual violence, and stalking used in the *NISVS* military report were aligned to closely match DoD definitions. "Contact sexual violence" in particular was aligned to the DoD definition of the range of crimes under the UCMJ constituting an adult sexual assault.

Some of the key findings of the survey are:

The risk of contact sexual violence for military and civilian women is the same, after controlling for age and marital status differences between these groups.

With few exceptions, the past-year and lifetime prevalence (occurrence) of IPV, sexual violence, and stalking in the civilian and military populations are quite similar, with no statistically significant differences.

Active-duty women were significantly less likely than civilian women to indicate that they experienced IPV in the three years prior to the survey.

Active-duty women were less likely to experience stalking than civilian women.

A deployment history appears to impact active-duty women's experience of IPV and sexual violence. Active-duty women with a deployment history had higher rates of IPV and sexual violence than women without a deployment history. These differences appeared in the past 3-year and lifetime prevalence rates, but were not present in the past-year prevalence rates. This suggests that IPV and sexual violence are problems that may develop over time for active-duty women who have been deployed.

HANDLING COMPLAINTS

Despite unprecedented attention and involvement from senior leadership, enhanced SAPR policies and training, and outreach to key stakeholders, sexual assault remains a persistent problem in the military. Current efforts to improve the Department's investigative and prosecutorial capabilities are important, but are not enough to solve this problem. Prevention-focused policies and initiatives are also necessary to achieve lasting cultural change. DoD SAPRO is working with the Military Services to implement initiatives that establish and foster a command climate in which bystanders are empowered to intervene in situations where there is a risk for sexual assault; sexist behavior and sexual assault are not condoned, tolerated, or ignored; victims are supported and do not fear retaliation for reporting; care is delivered; and offenders are held appropriately accountable for their crimes. Commanders and their leadership teams are critical to ensuring unit climates promote and enforce dignity, respect, and safety.

DoD SAPRO also plans to:

> promote initiatives that address sexual assault against male victims;
> host outreach meetings with external advocacy organizations and educational institutions to share prevention best practices; and
> develop standardized core competencies and learning objectives for a variety of SAPR trainings, including accession, annual refresher, and pre-deployment training, as well as professional military education.

Additionally, the Department will implement the requirement to provide an explanation of SAPR policies and resources to all service members at the time of (or within 14 duty days after) their initial entrance on active duty or into a duty status with a Reserve Component.

DEVELOPING SEXUAL ASSAULT
PREVENTION AND RESPONSE PROGRAMS

Sexual harassment prevention is a three-tier process. First, the organization must establish an organizational policy; secondly, provide adequate sexual harassment training; and lastly, develop the necessary tools for its employers (synonymous with commanders) to prevent harassment within the working environment. Employers who make the effort to prevent sexual harassment from occurring can benefit by avoiding a host of potential problems. Taking steps to prevent sexual harassment before it occurs benefits the organization in many practical ways as well.

An important prevention strategy includes conducting training on the following:

- what sexual harassment is and what it is not, from both legal and practical points of view;
- the difference between sexual harassment and inappropriate conduct, and why both need to be banned from the workplace;
- the types of sexual harassment and the implications for employer and person liability of each;
- how internal investigations are triggered and what happens during such investigations;
- the need for minimizing any discussion of sexual harassment situations, both formally and informally;
- the legal and organizational requirements for non-retaliation against those who raise sexual harassment concerns;
- the corporate options for post-investigation discipline and the factors that decision makers use in selecting that discipline;
- external charge mechanisms;
- what every supervisor and manager is expected to do in his or her own area to prevent sexual harassment from occurring, whether in terms of personal behavior, coworker relationships, or visitor conduct; and
- who the designated organizational person to receive reports of possible sexual harassment is, and the need for early reporting.

The U.S. Navy's SAPR Stand Down

The Navy's training program asks a number of questions to drive home the magnitude of the problem with data and what people think. The questions and scenarios are, however, applicable to all branches of the military.

QUESTION: When you hear about a sexual assault case, how often do you doubt the truthfulness of the victim's report and instead focus on the characteristics of the victim? What the victim was wearing, if the victim had been drinking, if the victim voluntarily invited the alleged offender to his or her own room?

What to listen for:

☐ The tendency to assume the report is false or that the victim is lying is not supported by the data.
☐ Victims of sexual assault are far more likely to have been assaulted and never tell anyone of the incident than they are to have never been assaulted and made a false report.

QUESTION: How often are you skeptical of an assault because you feel like you identify with the alleged perpetrator? "I know this guy." "He's a good guy." "He's a lot like me." "She would never do something like that." "He or she is a great Sailor."
What to listen for:

☐ Most victims know their perpetrators who are often described as "nice guys," difficult to distinguish from those you like and may respect.

QUESTION: When you think of sexual assault, how often do you think only of female victims?
What to listen for:

☐ There are additional stereotypes and myths that impact a man's ability to face their sexual assault and seek support or services, including:
  ☐ men are immune to victimization.
  ☐ men should be able to fight off attacks.
  ☐ men shouldn't express emotion.
★These are NOT true!
☐ According to the Navy's FY 2012 Annual Report to DoD, there were 425 Unrestricted Reports and 204 Restricted Reports of sexual assault made by female victims; 55 unrestricted reports and 37 restricted reports were made by male victims.
☐ Of those reported sexual assaults, 89 percent of victims were female and 11 percent of victims were male.

QUESTION: Preventing sexual assault is a leadership issue. By virtue of wearing the uniform, we're all leaders. What is your personal definition of leadership?

What to listen for:

☐ By example
☐ Walks the walk
☐ Respected and respectful
☐ Does the right thing when no one is watching
☐ Sets standards and keep standards

QUESTION: CNO asked us to refocus our efforts on sexual assault. Why would we begin by asking you about leadership? What's the connection?
What to listen for:

☐ It takes leadership and courage to confront shipmates and friends who are being abusive or pushing appropriate boundaries and limits.
☐ We need leadership from every one of us to refocus our attention on this very serious challenge.
☐ We lead in a variety of ways and the Navy needs Sailors to show the courage it takes to be leaders in preventing sexual assault.

QUESTION: What does everyone in the command think if you notice leadership is silent in the face of a vulgar e-mail or sexist comments?
What to listen for:

☐ Officer and enlisted leadership is essential.
☐ While most who laugh at an off-color joke or forward an inappropriate e-mail do not commit sexual assault—those who do commit this violence often mask and justify their behavior within climates where such behavior is condoned or ignored. Just as peers may provide inadvertent cover for offenders, they are also a very effective tool in both the prevention and response arenas. Emphasize the important role Sailors can play as active bystanders. Armed with basic education and training on resources and intervention strategies, they are a force multiplier.

QUESTION: What does Sexism look like?
What to listen for:

☐ Sexism relies on stereotypical gender roles and male dominance; subtle example—males continually restate what female members just stated.

☐ It reinforces men as protectors and providers, and males as having the greater power, authority, and physical strength; consequently, women must have less power, less authority, and less physical strength.

☐ It separates people because of their differences, regardless of gender; males that don't fit the mold of muscular and masculine are seen as inferior, and women who don't fit the mold as housewife and homemaker are seen as too dominant.

☐ Discussion regarding sexism should address situations involving male and female with a view toward acknowledging and eliminating behaviors and attitudes that disempower people.

☐ Sexism has an adverse effect on people's idea of what is worthwhile about them—it perpetuates stereotypes.

QUESTION: The military has been accused of moving too slowly on the issue of sexual assault in our ranks and there needs to be a greater sense of urgency in dealing with this problem. Without question, we are a male-dominated workforce. But by putting this problem in the box as a women's issue, do we diminish it? What role does sexism play in our everyday experiences—consider that 23 percent of the Navy's population might be having a different experience? The best examples are the gray ones.

What to consider:

☐ How do you talk to each other? Do you use first names, nicknames? Rank? Position? Does it matter if the person is male or female?

☐ Do you refer to men by their formal title and women by their first name?

☐ What about female officers? Do women do this to themselves by saying such things as "please, call me Joan"?

☐ Have you ever graciously opened the door for a woman to enter only to let it slam on the man directly behind her?

☐ Do you look to the men for answers regarding highly technical or arduous tasks?

☐ How does the language you use differ around men and women? Do you talk "down" to females?

☐ Do you double check or verify a woman's work with a man you believe to be technically competent?

☐ Are the tasks you assign or are assigned seen as "women's work" or a "man's job"? What effect does this have on who does the work?

The examples may seem trivial to some people, but it is this culture that allows offenses such as sexual assault to occur. Every individual is a valuable member of our Navy and should be treated with dignity and respect.

QUESTION: What is the Navy's definition of "sexual assault"?
What to listen for:

☐ Walking up to a shipmate and grabbing their genitals or breasts is NOT "horseplay"; it's a sexual assault!

☐ There is no informal resolution process for sexual assault.

☐ Uniform Code of Military Justice (Article 120) = a sexual act upon another person such as rape, sexual assault, aggravated sexual contact, and abusive sexual contact.

☐ "Sexual assault" is an umbrella term that includes both contact and penetration offenses.

☐ Offenses include the "good game" slaps (hits on the buttocks), the grabbing or touching of someone's genitals . . . all the way to violent rape.

☐ Uniform Code of Military Justice (Article 125) = forced engagement in unnatural carnal copulation with another person of the same sex or opposite sex or with an animal is guilty of sodomy; penetration, however slight, is sufficient to complete the offense.

☐ Uniform Code of Military Justice (Article 80) = an attempt to commit an offense even though failing to effect its commission, is an attempt to commit that offense.

QUESTION: What is the Navy's policy on sexual assault?
What to listen for:

☐ Sexual assault is completely unacceptable in the Navy; the ultimate goal is a command climate of gender respect where sexual assault is never tolerated and is completely eliminated.

☐ There is no single easy method to prevent sexual assault—it will require our sustained commitment—mentoring Sailors in decision-making; confronting alcohol issues; educating all Sailors about our shared responsibility as bystanders; and actively eradicating sexism and sexual harassment whenever encountered.

☐ Studies show that a coordinated response by a multidisciplinary approach improves a victim's experience as well as offender accountability.

GROUP ACTIVITY: *SEXUAL HARASSMENT VERSUS SEXUAL ASSAULT*

ASK: I'm going to read a statement, and I want you to tell me if it is "sexual assault" or "sexual harassment" and then tell me why:

1. Undressing a co-worker with your eyes in the workplace.
   - □ Answer: *Sexual harassment*. This can create a hostile or uncomfortable work environment.
2. Fondling a body part that would be covered by a swimsuit without consent.
   - □ Answer: *Sexual assault*. This is sexual contact; if it is unwanted, it is a sexual assault.
3. "Sexting" a co-worker or others who find the material offensive.
   - □ Answer: *Sexual harassment*. "Sexting" refers to sexually explicit text messages (text or images). This can create a hostile or uncomfortable work environment.

★★ IMPORTANT NOTE ★★

A lot of times we laugh and joke about these kinds of behaviors.

But if you look at the actions for what they really are—touching in sexual manner without permission—you'll realize that those actions constitute sexual assault.

Sexual assault is any unwanted intentional sexual contact.

QUESTION: What is consent?

What to listen for:

Consent is:
- □ Based on choice
- □ Active, not passive
- □ Talking about sex with your partner and how far you want it to go
- □ Knowing your partner wants you as much as you want them
- □ Listening and being listened to
- □ Giving permission without feeling pressured
- □ About open communication, caring, and respect
- □ Asking and hearing a yes
- □ Being on the same page as the person you're intimate with
- □ Engaging with each other and being clear about what you want
- □ Positive cooperation in the exercise of free will
- □ Talking about things you like, as well as being open about the things you don't like

☐ Setting your boundaries and only doing what you're comfortable with

☐ When both or all parties are fully conscious, mutually participating, and have positively and clearly communicated their intent

☐ Being able to say no at any time and that choice will be accepted and respected

QUESTION: So what is NOT consent?
What to listen for:

☐ Silence is not consent.

☐ You do not have consent if your partner is passed out.

☐ Intoxication is not consent.

☐ Alcohol can impair a person's ability to consent; alcohol use does not preclude the ability to give or receive consent, but having sexual contact or act with a person who has been drinking is legally risky.

☐ Fear is not consent.

☐ You do not obtain consent by pressuring someone, by threatening, coercing, or forcing someone.

QUESTION: If we were to create a continuum of sex similar to what the Continuum of Harm looks like, where would we draw the line between sex and then the sex being a crime? Let's go through some important questions to think and talk about. . . .
What to listen for:

☐ If someone says no then after more foreplay willingly has sex, then is that rape?

☐ What does it mean if someone comes to your room?

☐ What behaviors are there that suggest that someone wants to have sex?

☐ What about kissing while dancing?

☐ What about "grinding" on the dance floor?

☐ What about taking one's clothes off?

☐ So how do you know then that someone wants to have sex?

☐ What does "Playing the game" mean?

☐ What is the, "I don't think we should" routine?

☐ Where does the myth that "no" means "yes" come from?

☐ What does "hooking up" mean?

☐ How about "fooling around?" If it means different things to different people, then isn't it important to be precise?

GROUP ACTIVITY: *RISK REDUCTION*

GOAL: Show that the threat of sexual harassment and sexual assault is an omnipresent part of women's lives.

DIRECTIONS: IMPORTANT! Try not to vary from the step-by-step instructions when conducting this activity.

1. STATE: "Are men and women different? In society, do we have a habit of putting women in one box and men in another? For example—How many female warriors are there in the latest versions of the 'Call of Duty' or 'Halo' video games?"

2. Ask the questions posed below.

3. Record responses on chart paper or a dry erase board until ideas are exhausted.

PART 1 (*For the Men*)

ASK: "Men, tell me what you do on a daily basis to reduce the risk of being sexually assaulted." (Or you can clarify by saying, "What steps do you take every day to keep yourself safe from the threat of sexual assault?")

** IMPORTANT NOTE **

The men might have a hard time with this question and remain fairly silent. There might be a few glib responses and nervous laughter. They might say, "Well, I never really think about it." It is common for them to come up with NO actual responses to this question (if so, leave the page blank for the visual effect).

PART 2 (*For the Women*)

STATE: "Watch what happens when we ask the women in the room the same question."

ASK: "Women, tell me what you do on a daily basis to reduce the risk of being sexually assaulted." (Or you can clarify by saying, "What steps do you take every day to keep yourself safe from the threat of sexual assault?") *The list should be written unstructured to symbolize the overwhelmingness with the answers all over the place.*

Possible responses:

- "I never walk alone at night."
- "I sometimes dress down as not to call attention to myself."
- "I always carry a cell phone."
- "I go out with a group and come home with a group."
- "I never leave a drink unattended."

- "I carry a set of keys between my fingers as a weapon as I'm walk-ing."
- "I am trained in self-defense."
- "I lock my doors and windows."

** IMPORTANT NOTE **

Women will typically respond immediately; however, if you need to probe for answers, use the following questions:

- What do you do when going out to a bar?
- What do you do when walking home at night?
- Back in the day when we still had land lines, was there anything you would do regarding your phone listing in the telephone book or your recorded voice messages?
- Do you always have taxi money, a full tank of gas?
- What do you do when traveling alone?
- What do you do when in a car alone traveling or in a parking lot?

At this point you may have men contributing to the women's list. Insist upon hearing only from the women for the moment

** IMPORTANT NOTE **

Responses (if any) typically will not apply to preventing sexual assault. Be sure to ask: "Are you primarily doing that to prevent sexual assault or are you primarily concerned about other crimes?"

Men may become uncomfortable with the unevenness of the two lists and start building theirs up again.

Men and women might get defensive and relay that men are also the victim of sexual assault.

- Response: State, "You are absolutely correct: men can be and are also victims of sexual assault and this exercise in no way is trying to say otherwise."

Men might point out that during deployment there are some things that they will do to reduce their risk of being assaulted. Examples of this might be hyper-vigilance at night alone or in the shower.

- Response: State, "It may be correct that during deployment, the rates of victimization for men regarding sexual assault go up and conversely, so do rates of victimization for women. Think about that feeling of hyper-vigilance you are describing, men, in experiences during deployment. Now imagine feeling that way every day of your life."

Men might also clarify that they might not protect themselves specifi-cally from sexual assault, but that they do take steps to protect themselves from crimes like mugging, assault, or hate crimes.

- Response: State, "Women also take steps to protect themselves from those crimes. A significant difference between men and women regarding these crimes is that the underlying threat for women with these crimes is sexual assault."

PART 3 (*For All*)

ASK: "What do you notice about the two lists?"

Possible responses:

- Women have a lot more rules they have to follow.

- Men didn't realize how much more women are on guard all the time.

- Women are shocked when they realize how many of these rules they instinctively follow.

- Frustration by both men and women that this is the way it is.

ASK: "How do these make you feel?"

** IMPORTANT NOTE **

Understand the following points:

Typically, the men's list is limited to less than 2-3 responses while the women's list is usually so full that the chart paper is almost unreadable.

The practices women outlined are not only what women do every day, but what they are EXPECTED to do, and if they don't, they are questioned and criticized for not practicing risk reduction.

If women are not carefully practicing these risk-reduction techniques, they are often blamed for the crimes committed against them.

It's okay that men and women are different. It needs to be openly acknowledged in order to encourage community involvement and drive culture change.

QUESTION: Historically, risk reduction has been the major prevention effort to reduce sexual assault and harassment in both the civilian and military communities. So if we've really got a problem, why don't we focus more on sexual assault risk reduction?

What to listen for:

☐ The reality is that risk reduction is not reducing the number of incidents.

☐ We have shipmates assaulting other shipmates—people you know and trust, not typically the stranger in a ski mask.

☐ The reality is that focusing only on the victim is short sighted— it does not stop the perpetrator from trying again, and again, and again.

☐ Risk reduction puts most of the focus on women and sexual assault is a gender-neutral offense.

☐ It does not provide support for survivors because people often question what the survivor did or didn't do.

☐ To end sexual assault and harassment, we need to start examining the attitudes, beliefs, and actions that support a rape culture.

QUESTION: So how does sexual assault prevention differ from risk reduction?

What to listen for:

☐ It seeks to stop the behavior before it happens by recognizing that there is only ONE person truly capable of preventing a sexual assault 100 percent of the time: the offender.

☐ Like Bystander Intervention, sexual assault prevention encourages community involvement and cultural change.

☐ Rather than blaming victims, prevention strategies hold the perpetrators of sexual violence responsible.

☐ We must change a culture that allows perpetrators of sexual assault to fly under the radar undetected, unchallenged, and unaccountable.

☐ Encouraging Bystander Intervention strategies, focusing our efforts on prevention instead of risk reduction, and holding perpetrators appropriately accountable are the building blocks to cultural change.

QUESTION: What does "integrity" really mean? How can we recognize the moral gravity of each personal and professional decision?

What to listen for:

☐ Does this decision respect laws, rules, and standards of conduct?

☐ Does this decision reflect the Navy's core values of honor, courage, and commitment?

☐ Does this decision contribute to a constructive outcome for me and others?

☐ Does this decision safely and legally contribute to mission readiness and completion?

☐ Individuals are responsible for the actions they take, as well as the ones they do not.

☐ Each of us is an ambassador for our command, the Navy, and our country.

QUESTION: Doing the right thing when no one is looking also means managing the freedom to do whatever you want. A lot of us came into the Navy straight from high school, where our freedoms were still regulated by our parents. Even so, now we're all regulated by Navy policy and rules and regulations. Why is it that when left to our own choices some of us begin to set and drift, eventually crossing the line into possible criminal activity? What is so difficult about personal responsibility and making the right choice?

What to listen for:

- ☐ I never had the chance to "test the waters" before stepping into an organization with such a high moral code.
- ☐ It's difficult to stop myself when I'm having fun.

QUESTION: Where's your red line? We all have a line to mark the limits of our own personal standards of behavior and insist it's a line we would never cross. Is yours a permanent red line? Does it move as a matter of convenience to fit a situation? Does it continue to move as you progress in rank and/or stature? Is your line at the same spot as others? And what happens when you cross the line—can you go back?

What to listen for:

- ☐ Situational boundaries when hard red lines should exist.
- ☐ Think about driving down a long stretch of empty back road and you come to a red light in the middle of nowhere. You stop and look both ways and no traffic is in sight for miles. Do you wait for the light to turn green or do you proceed through the light in order to shorten your travel time? Will your red line move in this situation?
- ☐ Where is our line when we want to fit in with the team and either participate in the crude jokes or be complacent when it comes to objecting?

DECISION-MAKING in Action:

- ☐ *A Sailor is faced with a choice to accurately report less-than-high performance on a damage control (DC) drill, or "gun deck" the information for the sake of appearance. She chooses to report accurately, reasoning that the importance of DC capability aboard her ship is vital to everyone's wellbeing.*

☐ *A junior officer (JO) recognizes that his Department Head is on the verge of accepting an invitation from a contractor that may violate the Joint Ethics Regulation. Some of his fellow JOs pressure him to keep silent about the issue and not rock the boat. Instead, he chooses to speak with his Department Head about his concerns, and points out the possible ethical risk.*

QUESTION: The choice to act requires decision. Bystander Intervention is a primary component of sexual assault prevention. Why is it so imperative that we step up and step in when we see a shipmate heading down a potentially dangerous path?
What to listen for:

☐ We will never break the cycle of harm if we don't step up and step in.
☐ It's hard to intervene—what if I'm wrong?
☐ Don't want to appear stupid.

QUESTION: It's about choice. Sexual activity is a personal choice. What kind of decisions are Sailors faced with in terms of sexuality, especially during extended deployments?
What to listen for:

☐ Mission first, shipmates always.
☐ The discussion needs to include eliminating the behavior of looking at fellow Sailors as an opportunity for sexual gratification.
☐ Discuss personal discipline around sexual behaviors.

QUESTION: Drinking is a personal choice. What kind of decisions are Sailors faced with in terms of drinking?
What to listen for:

☐ It can lower inhibitions/cloud judgment.
☐ It can impact a person's ability to consent.
☐ It can impede the judgment of bystanders.

QUESTION: The fact is that there are Service members who drink alcohol. However, some Sailors don't understand the effects of their alcohol use and end up making choices that result in negative outcomes; in addition, they open themselves up to increased risk. What does responsible drinking really mean? How much is too much?

What to listen for:

- ☐ Know your limits.
- ☐ Drink in moderation.
- ☐ Don't drink underage—underage drinking is illegal and a violation of the UCMJ.
- ☐ Command specific policy on responsible alcohol use, example "0013":
  - ☐ Zero underage drinking
  - ☐ Zero drinking and driving
  - ☐ One drink per hour
  - ☐ No more than three drinks per night

QUESTION: How often do you assume that an alleged sexual assault is more likely to be an encounter between well-intentioned individuals who simply had regrets the next day?

What to listen for:

- ☐ Every case stands alone.
- ☐ Common tactics used to commit the assault include: ignoring victims' efforts to communicate, incapacitating them with alcohol or drugs, physical force, or threats.
- ☐ Every case must be thoroughly investigated by law enforcement so that the facts relevant to that case can be determined; then, and only then, after you thoroughly review the case, can you reach a disposition decision that is fair to both the victim and alleged perpetrator in that individual case.
- ☐ The prime factor behind a sexual encounter not being seen as sexual assault is the exchange of clearly communicated consent from both or all parties.
- ☐ In the absence of clear consent, a case could be made for sexual assault.

QUESTION: Is there such a thing as situational offenders of sexual assault? Someone who takes advantage of the right combination of circumstances "to get some sex?" For example, our alleged subject has a lack of impulse control, no self-discipline, and poor sexual boundaries; he goes and drinks too much alcohol (irresponsible drinking), and then discovers a victim of opportunity (a fellow Sailor who is significantly drunk). This creates the potential for a situation that can possibly lead to sexual assault. What are your thoughts on Navy's assaults—do you think they are committed by situational offenders? How do we prevent those?

What to listen for:

☐ Sailors don't take advantage of fellow sailors.
☐ No premeditation, just a matter of circumstance.
☐ Situation lent itself to low risk, high reward.
☐ Lack of consent in a situation like this.
☐ Bystander intervention would protect BOTH sailors.

QUESTION: It is imperative that every man and woman has consent prior to sexual intimacy—this applies to both non-married and married partners. Consent is a decision. Consent is essential. So as we discussed before, what do you do to get consent?

What to listen for:

☐ ASK!
☐ "No" means no.
☐ "Not now" means no.
☐ "I don't know if I want to" means no.
☐ Hearing no does not mean slow down; it means stop.
☐ "I had too much to drink" means no.
☐ "I'm not sure" means no.
☐ "I'm scared" means no.
☐ Sex without consent is a crime.
☐ Only "yes" means yes.

QUESTION: So how do you ask for consent?
What to listen for:

☐ Can I kiss you?
☐ Is this okay?
☐ Are you comfortable with this?
☐ What would you like me to do?
☐ Do you like it when I do this?
☐ Do you want to have sex?
☐ Notice in this section how often "this," "there," etc., are used. Why not ask—can I touch your breast? If you can't be explicit, are you ready for sex?

☐ It is okay to openly acknowledge that you and your partner have sexual desires.

☐ It's important for you to respect yourself and your partner and accept their beliefs and their values.

QUESTION: What are the official reporting options available to a victim of sexual assault?

What to listen for:

☐ Unrestricted Report

A process used by an individual to disclose, without requesting Restricted Reporting, that he or she is the victim of a sexual assault. Under these circumstances, the victim's report to the SARC, healthcare personnel, a victim advocate, command authorities, NCIS, local law enforcement, a chaplain, judge advocate, or other persons are reportable to law enforcement and may be used to initiate the official investigation process.

☐ Restricted Report

A process used by an eligible individual to report or disclose that he or she is the victim of a sexual assault to specified officials on a requested confidential basis. Under these circumstances, the victim's report and any details provided to the SARC, SAPR VA, or healthcare personnel constitute a Restricted Report. Such a report to these personnel as well as to a legal assistance attorney or chaplain will not be reported to law enforcement to initiate an official investigation.

☐ When a victim elects to remain silent the allegation is never investigated; the subject is never held accountable and the event remains a secret. Perpetrators thrive on secrecy and actually target their victims based on the belief that the victim will keep the secret.

** CIVILIAN PERSONNEL ONLY **

☐ In most cases, if you're a civilian, you are only eligible to make an Unrestricted Report of sexual assault. Certainly there are SARCs and VAs who can help, but by policy, Restricted Reports are not an option. The SARC and SAPR VA are available resources for emergent support and can assist you. (For additional civilian eligibility information, see DODI 6495.02.)

QUESTION: What do you think prevents or would prevent victims from reporting within our command?

What to listen for:

- ☐ This question is often asked out of well-intentioned frustration at feeling helpless to act in the fact of an assault.
- ☐ The reality is that reasons victims give for not reporting include things within a command's reach to address, including:
  - ☐ Did not want superiors to know
  - ☐ Fear of being treated badly if they report
  - ☐ Concern for protecting their identity
  - ☐ Did not trust the reporting process
  - ☐ Afraid of retaliation
  - ☐ Thought nothing would be done
  - ☐ Perception they could handle it on their own
- ☐ The ultimate responsibility resides with the command to create a safe environment where reporting is encouraged.
- ☐ Note what is being communicated within the command that is contributing to barriers to report and address them.
- ☐ Of the Navy commands that had answered the required sexual assault questions on the DEOCS between 01 March and 21 May 2013:
  - ☐ 45 percent of men and 57 percent of women perceived stigma, shame, and fear as barriers to reporting sexual assault.
  - ☐ 29 percent of men and 40 percent of women feared re-victimization if they reported.
  - ☐ 40 percent of men and 26 percent of women reported no barriers to reporting sexual assault.

QUESTION: Some victims choose not to come forward, or choose to file a Restricted rather than an Unrestricted Report. How can we increase a climate of victim confidence associated with reporting so that victims trust their command and feel supported to report and participate in the investigation and adjudication process?

What to listen for:

- ☐ Leverage leadership at all levels, particularly those most directly connected with the target, most vulnerable audience.
- ☐ Create community-empowered bystander intervention.
- ☐ Train first responders.

☐ Address sexual assault reporting options and reducing stigma in awareness training at all levels.

☐ Execute SAPR initiatives at the deck plate level.

☐ Behave in a way that is transparent to the people we have the privilege of leading.

☐ Conduct a SAPR Response drill to ensure all parts of the command system function as they are meant to function.

QUESTION: Based on today's discussions, how might our biases be impacting the prevention and response efforts of this command?

What to listen for:

☐ The messages we communicate formally and informally can decrease victim blaming, increase the scrutiny of repeat offenders, and increase the reporting and help-seeking behaviors of victims.

☐ Eliminating sexual harassment and sexual violence is everyone's responsibility.

☐ Your words and actions, or lack thereof, set the deciding tone.

☐ Identifying potential liabilities in terms or misinformation or personal biases is a crucial first step.

QUESTION: SAPR-L and SAPR-F are both titled "TAKE THE HELM"—Why do you think that is?

What to listen for:

☐ It is up to all of us E-1 to O-10 to step up and step in when we see something wrong.

☐ CNO states that each of us needs to be the first line of defense.

☐ We all need to refocus, take charge of this problem, and steer it in the right direction.

☐ Success will only be achieved with an all-hands, top-to-bottom, concerted effort to eliminate sexual assault from our ranks.

ACROSS-THE-BOARD POLICIES

In May 2013 the secretary of defense directed the secretaries of the Military Departments, chairman of the Joint Chiefs of Staff, under secretary of defense for personnel and readiness, chiefs of the Military Services, chief of the National Guard Bureau, and general counsel of the Department of

Defense to implement the 2013 SAPR Strategic Plan "to achieve unity of effort and purpose across the Department."

He also ordered immediate implementation of the following measures "to strengthen our sexual assault prevention and response programs, specifically addressing accountability, command climate and victim advocacy."

- Enhancing Commander Accountability: To further enhance command accountability, the Service Chiefs, through their respective Secretaries of the Military Departments, will develop methods to assess the performance of military commanders in establishing command climates of dignity and respect and incorporating SAPR prevention and victim care principles in their commands, and hold them accountable. Report your methods tome through USD (P&R) by November 1, 2013.
- Improving Response and Victim Treatment: To improve overall victim care and trust in the chain of command, increase reporting, and reduce the possibility of ostracizing victims, the Secretaries of the Military Departments will implement and monitor methods to improve victim treatment by their peers, co-workers, and chains of command. Solicit victim input in the development of these methods. Report your methods to me through USD (P&R) by November 1, 2013.
- Assessing Military Justice Systems: To ensure a timely and independent assessment of the systems used to investigate, prosecute, and adjudicate crimes involving adult sexual assault and related offenses assessment of military justice systems, I call upon the panel established under Section 576 of the FY13 National Defense Authorization Act to accelerate its review and provide final recommendations to me within 12 months of the panel's first meeting.
- Enhancing Commander Accountability: To enhance accountability and improve insight into subordinate command climate, the USD (P&R) shall require that the results of FY13 National Defense Authorization Act-mandated annual command climate surveys will now also be provided to the next level up in the chain of command. Implement this provision not later than July 31, 2013.
- Ensuring Safety: To ensure the awareness and safety of our newest and aspiring Service members, the Secretaries of the Military Departments will improve the effectiveness of sexual assault prevention and response programs in recruiting organizations, Military Entrance Processing Stations, and the Reserve Officer Training Corps. These

assessments will include: 1) the selection, SAPR training, and oversight of recruiters; 2) the dissemination of SAPR program information to potential and actual recruits; and 3) the prevention and education programs in ROTC environments and curricula. Report your findings to me through USD (P&R) by September 30, 2013.

- Ensuring Appropriate Command Climate: To ensure DoD facilities promote an environment of dignity and respect and are free from materials that create a degrading or offensive work environment, DoD component heads will direct comprehensive and regular visual inspections of all DoD workplaces, to include military academies, by July 1, 2013. The Air Force conducted such an inspection in FY13 and will therefore only report the findings and actions taken from that previously conducted inspection. Report your findings to me through USD (P&R) by July 31, 2013.

- Enhancing Commander Accountability: To further enhance command accountability, the Service Chiefs, through their respective Secretaries of the Military Departments, will develop methods to assess the performance of military commanders in establishing command climates of dignity and respect and incorporating SAPR prevention and victim care principles in their commands, and hold them accountable. Report your methods to me through USD (P&R) by November 1, 2013.

- Improving Response and Victim Treatment: To improve overall victim care and trust in the chain of command, increase reporting, and reduce the possibility of ostracizing victims, the Secretaries of the Military Departments will implement and monitor methods to improve victim treatment by their peers, co-workers, and chains of command. Solicit victim input in the development of these methods. Report your methods to me through USD (P&R) by November 1, 2013.

- Assessing Military Justice Systems: To ensure a timely and independent assessment of the systems used to investigate, prosecute, and adjudicate crimes involving adult sexual assault and related offenses assessment of military justice systems, I call upon the panel established under Section 576 of the FY13 National Defense Authorization Act to accelerate its review and provide final recommendations to me within 12 months of the panel's first meeting.

- Enhancing Commander Accountability: To enhance accountability and improve insight into subordinate command climate, the USD (P&R) shall require that the results of FY13 National Defense Authorization Act-mandated annual command climate surveys will now also be provided to the next level up in the chain of command. Implement this provision not later than July 31, 2013.

- Ensuring Safety: To ensure the awareness and safety of our newest and aspiring Service members, the Secretaries of the Military Departments will improve the effectiveness of sexual assault prevention and response programs in recruiting organizations, Military Entrance Processing Stations, and the Reserve Officer Training Corps. These assessments will include: 1) the selection, SAPR training, and oversight of recruiters; 2) the dissemination of SAPR program information to potential and actual recruits; and 3) the prevention and education programs in ROTC environments and curricula. Report your findings to me through USD (P&R) by September 30, 2013.
- Ensuring Appropriate Command Climate: To ensure DoD facilities promote an environment of dignity and respect and are free from materials that create a degrading or offensive work environment, DoD component heads will direct comprehensive and regular visual inspections of all DoD workplaces, to include military academies, by July 1, 2013. The Air Force conducted such an inspection in FY13 and will therefore only report the findings and actions taken from that previously conducted inspection. Report your findings to me through USD (P&R) by July 31, 2013.
- Enhancing Commander Accountability: To further enhance command accountability, the Service Chiefs, through their respective Secretaries of the Military Departments, will develop methods to assess the performance of military commanders in establishing command climates of dignity and respect and incorporating SAPR prevention and victim care principles in their commands, and hold them accountable.
- Improving Response and Victim Treatment: To improve overall victim care and trust in the chain of command, increase reporting, and reduce the possibility of ostracizing victims, the Secretaries of the Military Departments will implement and monitor methods to improve victim treatment by their peers, co-workers, and chains of command. Solicit victim input in the development of these methods.
- Assessing Military Justice Systems: To ensure a timely and independent assessment of the systems used to investigate, prosecute, and adjudicate crimes involving adult sexual assault and related offenses assessment of military justice systems, I call upon the panel

established under Section 576 of the FY13 National Defense Authorization Act to accelerate its review and provide final recommendations to me within 12 months of the panel's first meeting.

- Enhancing Commander Accountability: To enhance accountability and improve insight into subordinate command climate, the USD (P&R) shall require that the results of FY13 National Defense Authorization Act-mandated annual command climate surveys will now also be provided to the next level up in the chain of command. Implement this provision not later than July 31, 2013.
- Ensuring Safety: To ensure the awareness and safety of our newest and aspiring Service members, the Secretaries of the Military Departments will improve the effectiveness of sexual assault prevention and response programs in recruiting organizations, Military Entrance Processing Stations, and the Reserve Officer Training Corps. These assessments will include: 1) the selection, SAPR training, and oversight of recruiters; 2) the dissemination of SAPR program information to potential and actual recruits; and 3) the prevention and education programs in ROTC environments and curricula.
- Ensuring Appropriate Command Climate: To ensure DoD facilities promote an environment of dignity and respect and are free from materials that create a degrading or offensive work environment, DoD component heads will direct comprehensive and regular visual inspections of all DoD workplaces, to include military academies, by July 1, 2013. The Air Force conducted such an inspection in FY13 and will therefore only report the findings and actions taken from that previously conducted inspection.

Finally, to enhance the administration of military justice, I am directing the DoD Acting General Counsel to take the following actions:

- Ensuring Victim's Rights: Develop a method, in coordination with the Joint Service Committee (JSC) on Military Justice, to incorporate the rights afforded to victims through the Crime Victims' Rights Act into military justice practice, to the extent appropriate.
- Improving Victim's Counsel: Evaluate the Air Force Special Victims Counsel pilot program and other approaches to ensure that victims of sexual assault are provided the advice and assistance they need to understand their rights and to feel confident in the military justice system.

"The Department needs to be a national leader in preventing and responding to sexual assault. We are committed to lead the daughters and sons of the American people with the values of our honorable profession and to ensure they serve in an environment that is free from sexual assault and protects the dignity and respect of every Service member. These initiatives and plans, in addition to our on-going efforts, provide a roadmap for this Department to establish the enduring culture that is required of our profession of arms."

VICTIM ADVOCACY PROGRAMS

Victims' use of advocacy services is optional; however, commanders must ensure that victims have access to a well-coordinated, highly responsive sexual assault victim advocacy program that is available 24 hours per day, 7 days per week both in the garrison and in a deployed environment.

a. There are three echelons of sexual assault victim advocates in the Army's program in garrison:
   1. The installation SARC is responsible for coordinating the local implementation of the program.
   2. Installation victim advocates (IVA) work directly with the installation SARC, victims of sexual assault, unit victim advocates, and other installation response agencies.
   3. UVAs are soldiers who are trained to provide limited victim advocacy as a collateral duty.

b. In a deployed environment, there are two echelons of victim advocates:
   1. Deployable SARCs are soldiers trained and responsible for coordinating the Sexual Assault Prevention and Response Program as a collateral duty in a specified area of a deployed theater.
   2. There is one deployable SARC at each brigade/unit of action and higher echelon.
   3. UVAs are soldiers trained to provide victim advocacy as a collateral duty. There are two UVAs for each battalion-sized unit.

RESOURCES

SAMPLE MEMORANDUM OF UNDERSTANDING

SAMPLE
MOU Between
(INSTALLATION) Installation Law Enforcement Office and
(CITY, COUNTY, or STATE) Law Enforcement Agency
(Consult with the local Staff Judge Advocate and Agreements Manager before completing)

1. PURPOSE: To establish written procedures concerning the exchange of information, case investigation, cases involving civilian alleged offenders, jurisdiction, and coordination of efforts and assets between the (INSTALLATION) Installation Law Enforcement Office and (CITY, COUNTY, or STATE) Law Enforcement Agency in sexual assault cases involving an active duty Service member.

2. GENERAL: This MOU does not create additional jurisdiction or limit or modify existing jurisdiction vested in the parties. This MOU is intended exclusively to provide guidance and documents an agreement for general support between the (INSTALLATION) Installation Law Enforcement Office and (CITY, COUNTY, or STATE) Law Enforcement Agency. Nothing contained herein creates or extends any right, privilege, or benefit to any person or entity. (See DoD Directive 5400.11 (Reference (ah)). As used herein, the term "Service member" refers to an active duty Service member, Military Service Academy cadet or midshipmen, or National Guard or Reserve Service member when performing active service and inactive duty training (as defined in section 101(d)(3) of Reference (a)) or a member of

the Coast Guard or Coast Guard Reserve (when the Coast Guard is operating as a service in the Navy). A. [INSERT PARAGRAPH HERE DEFINING RESPONSE AND INVESTIGATION JURISDICTION FOR THE (INSTALLATION) INSTALLATION LAW ENFORCEMENT OFFICE AND (CITY, COUNTY, OR STATE) LAW ENFORCEMENT AGENCY.]

3. RESPONSIBILITIES:

A. The (CITY, COUNTY, or STATE) Law Enforcement Agency agrees to perform the following actions:

(1) When responding to or investigating sexual assault cases, the (CITY, COUNTY, or STATE) Law Enforcement Agency shall ascertain whether the alleged offender is a Service member. If the alleged offender is a Service member, the responding officer(s) shall note on the top of the incident/investigation report "Copy to the (INSTALLATION) Installation Law Enforcement" and the designated Records personnel shall ensure the copy is forwarded.

(2) When responding to or investigating sexual assault cases, the (CITY, COUNTY, or STATE) Law Enforcement Agency shall ascertain whether the victim is a Service member. If the victim is a Service member, the responding officer(s) shall seek the victim's consent to forward a copy of the incident/investigation report to the (INSTALLATION) Law Enforcement Office so that it can be provided to the victim's commander. If the victim so consents, the responding officer(s) shall note on the top of the incident/investigation report "Copy to the (INSTALLATION) Installation Law Enforcement Office" and the designated Records personnel shall ensure the copy is forwarded. If the victim does not consent, the responding officer(s) shall note in the body of the incident/investigation report that the victim did not consent to forwarding the report to the Installation Law Enforcement Office and shall not direct Records personnel to forward the report, but the report shall be provided to the Installation Sexual Assault Response Coordinator.

(3) When responding to or investigating sexual assault cases, and the (CITY, COUNTY, or STATE) Law Enforcement Agency ascertains that the alleged offender and the victim are both Service members, the responding officer(s) shall seek the victim's consent to forward a copy of the incident/investigation report

to the (INSTALLATION) Law Enforcement Office so that it can be provided to the victim's commander. If the victim so consents, the responding officer(s) shall note on the top of the incident/investigation report "Copy to the (INSTALLATION) Installation Law Enforcement Office" and the designated Records personnel shall ensure the copy is forwarded. If the victim does not consent, the responding officer(s) shall note in the body of the incident/investigation report that the victim did not consent to forwarding the report to the Installation Law Enforcement Office and shall not direct Records personnel to forward the report, but the report shall be provided to the Installation Sexual Assault Response Coordinator.

(4) When the (CITY, COUNTY, or STATE) Law Enforcement Agency receives a copy of a temporary or permanent civil protection order (CPO) issued by a court of competent jurisdiction, the responding officer(s) shall ascertain whether the alleged offender is an active duty Service member. If the alleged offender is active duty, the responding officer(s) shall note on the top of the CPO "Copy to the (INSTALLATION) Installation Law Enforcement Office" and the designated Records personnel shall ensure the copy is forwarded. [THIS PARAGRAPH MAY NOT BE NECESSARY IF THE INSTALLATION HAS AN MOU WITH THE LOCAL COURT SPECIFYING THAT THE COURT SHALL FORWARD COPIES OF SUCH CPOS TO THE INSTALLATION.]

(5) When the (CITY, COUNTY, or STATE) Law Enforcement Agency receives a copy of a temporary or permanent CPO, the responding officer(s) shall ascertain whether the victim is a Service member. If the victim is a Service member, the responding officer(s) shall seek the victim's consent to forward a copy of the CPO to the (INSTALLATION) Installation Law Enforcement Office. If the victim so consents, the responding officer(s) shall note on the top of the CPO "Copy to the (INSTALLATION) Installation Law Enforcement Office" and the designated Records personnel shall ensure the copy is forwarded. If the victim does not consent, the responding officer(s) shall not request that a copy of the CPO be forwarded to the Installation Law Enforcement Office.

(6) The (CITY, COUNTY, or STATE) Law Enforcement Agency shall designate an employee from Records who shall be directly responsible for forwarding copies of incident/investigation reports and CPOs to the (INSTALLATION) Installation Law Enforcement Office when directed to do so by notations at the top of the reports or CPOs. The (CITY, COUNTY, or STATE) Law Enforcement Agency employee shall also be responsible for receiving and processing of MPOs forwarded from the (INSTALLATION) Installation Law Enforcement Office.

(7) When the (CITY, COUNTY, or STATE) Law Enforcement Agency becomes aware of a violation of a term or provision of an MPO, the responding officer(s) shall notify the designated representative from the (INSTALLATION) Installation Law Enforcement Office of the violation.

(8) The (CITY, COUNTY, or STATE) Law Enforcement Agency shall provide the (INSTALLATION) Installation Law Enforcement Office with an area for Installation Law Enforcement investigators to conduct interviews of Service members who are involved in sexual assault incidents.

(9) The (INSTALLATION) Installation Law Enforcement office shall, when appropriate, conduct joint investigations with the (CITY, COUNTY, or STATE) Law Enforcement Agency if incidents of sexual assault involve Service members.

(10) When the victim in a sexual assault incident has been identified as a Service member, the (CITY, COUNTY, or STATE) Law Enforcement Agency responding officer(s) shall provide the victim with basic information, acquired from the Installation Law Enforcement Office (below) about installation resources available to sexual assault victims.

(11) As new law enforcement officers begin duty with the (CITY, COUNTY, or STATE) Law Enforcement Agency, their immediate supervisor shall provide them with copies of this MOU and basic instruction for effectuating the provisions of this MOU.

B. The (INSTALLATION) Installation Law Enforcement Office agrees to perform the following actions:

(1) The (INSTALLATION) Installation Law Enforcement Office shall designate an individual to act as liaison to the (CITY, COUNTY, or STATE) Law Enforcement Agency and to re-

ceive copies of incident/investigation reports stemming from an incident occurring off of the installation and CPOs involving Service members.

(2) Upon receipt of a copy of an incident/investigation report stemming from incidents occurring off of the installation or a CPO involving a Service member, the (INSTALLATION) Installation Law Enforcement Office shall immediately notify the Service member's Command.

(3) When the (INSTALLATION) Installation Law Enforcement Office receives a copy of an MPO from a Service member's Command, and if that Service member is living off of the installation, the (INSTALLATION) Installation Law Enforcement office shall forward a copy of the MPO to the (CITY, COUNTY, or STATE) Law Enforcement Agency with jurisdiction over the area in which the Service member resides.

(4) The (INSTALLATION) Installation Law Enforcement Office shall provide the (CITY, STATE, OR COUNTY) Police Department with an area for Police Department officers or investigators to conduct interviews of Service members who are involved in sexual assault incidents.

(5) The (INSTALLATION) Installation Law Enforcement office shall, when appropriate, conduct joint investigations with the (CITY, COUNTY, or STATE) Law Enforcement Agency if incidents of sexual assault involve Service members.

(6) The (INSTALLATION) Installation Law Enforcement Office shall assist the (CITY, COUNTY, or STATE) Law Enforcement Agency when investigating cases that occurred off base by providing information such as medical records, Military Service records, and incident/investigation reports from incidents occurring under the jurisdiction of the Installation Law Enforcement Office in accordance with the provisions of Section 552a of Reference (ab) and Reference (ac).

(7) The (INSTALLATION) Installation Law Enforcement Office shall provide the (CITY, COUNTY, or STATE) Law Enforcement Agency with basic information, in the form of quick reference cards or brochures, about installation resources available to sexual assault victims.

(8) [INSERT A PARAGRAPH HERE STATING PROPER INSTALLATION PROCEDURE FOR RESPONDING TO SEXUAL ASSAULT INCIDENTS OCCURRING ON THE INSTALLATION INVOLVING CIVILIAN ALLEGED OFFENDERS.]

(9) As new personnel begin duty with the (INSTALLATION) Installation Law Enforcement office, their immediate supervisor shall provide them with copies of this MOU and basic instructions on effectuating the provisions of this MOU.

4. EFFECTIVE ADMINISTRATION AND EXECUTION OF THIS MOU:
   A. This MOU shall be reviewed annually and shall remain in full force and effect until specifically abrogated by one of the parties to this agreement with 60 days written notice to the other party.
   B. Effective execution of this agreement can only be achieved through continuing communication and dialogue between the parties. It is the intent of this MOU that channels of communication shall be used to resolve questions, misunderstandings, or complaints that may arise that are not specifically addressed in this MOU.
   C. Personnel from the (INSTALLATION) Installation Law Enforcement Office and from the (CITY, COUNTY, or STATE) Law Enforcement Agency shall meet, as necessary and appropriate, to discuss open cases involving Service members and to share information regarding reciprocal investigations.
   D. The primary POC for this agreement is (INSTALLATION POC NAME; OFFICE OR ACTIVITY NAME, STREET ADDRESS, CITY, STATE, ZIP CODE, PHONE NUMBER, ORGANIZATIONAL EMAIL).

2012 SERVICE ACADEMY GENDER RELATIONS SURVEY

U.S. Military Academy

Overall, 10.7% of women and 1.7% of men indicated they experienced unwanted sexual contact in 2012. The percentage of women was higher in 2012 than in 2010 and no change for men. Of the 10.7% of women who indicated experiencing unwanted sexual contact, 44% (19 percentage points higher than 2010) indicated they experienced unwanted sexual touching only. Twenty-four % (15 percentage points lower than 2010) indicated the incident included attempted sex, with or without sexual touching; and 30% (unchanged from 2010) indicated they experienced completed sex, with or without sexual touching and/or attempted sex.

Unwanted Sexual Contact Details. Of the 10.7% of women who indicated experiencing unwanted sexual contact, nearly all (95%—3 percentage points lower than 2010) identified the offender as male, and most (82%—10 percentage points lower than 2010) indicated the offender was a fellow cadet.

Forty-six percent indicated alcohol and/or drugs were involved and 11% indicated threats and physical force were used (both unchanged from 2010). Nineteen percent (unchanged from 2010) indicated they reported the incident to a military authority or organization. The main reasons those women chose to report the incident were: it was the right thing to do (82%), to stop the offender from hurting others (73%), to stop the offender from hurting them again (65%), and to seek help dealing with an emotional incident (65%). The main reasons women chose not to report the incident were: they thought it was not important enough to report (75%—19 percentage points higher than 2010), they did not want people gossiping about them (74%—unchanged from 2010), and they did not want anyone to know (70%—8 percentage points higher than 2010).

Prior Unwanted Sexual Contact. Students were asked to indicate if they experienced any of the unwanted sexual contact behaviors prior to entering the Academy. The prior experience rate was 16.4% for women and 3.7% for men.

Unwanted Gender-Related Behaviors. Forty-nine percent of women and 8% of men indicated experiencing sexual harassment in 2012 (both unchanged from 2010). Eighty-two percent of women (2 percentage points lower than 2010) and 43% of men (unchanged from 2010) indicated experiencing crude/offensive behavior. Fifty-two percent of women (5 percentage points lower than 2010) and 12% of men (unchanged from 2010) indicated experiencing unwanted sexual attention. Seventeen percent of women (3 percentage points lower than 2010) and 4% of men (unchanged from 2010) indicated experiencing sexual coercion. Ninety-one percent of women (3 percentage points lower than 2010) and 33% of men (unchanged from 2010) indicated experiencing sexist behavior.

Unwanted Gender-Related Behavior Details. Ninety-three percent of women and 51% of men indicated experiencing one or more of the unwanted gender-related behaviors (i.e., crude/offensive behavior, unwanted sexual attention, sexual coercion, sexist behavior) in 2012. Of those, the majority of women (85%—4 percentage points higher than 2010) and men (67%—unchanged from 2010) identified the offender as a fellow cadet. Nine percent of women and 2% of men discussed the situation with a military authority or organization (both unchanged from 2010).

Stalking. Few women (4.4%—1.2 percentage points lower than 2010) and men (0.2%—unchanged from 2010) indicated that they experienced stalking-related behaviors that caused them fear of physical harm or sexual assault (the requirement to meet the legal definition of stalking).

U.S. Naval Academy

Unwanted Sexual Contact. Overall, 15.1% of women and 2.6% of men indicated they experienced unwanted sexual contact in 2012. There were no changes in the percentages of women or men in 2012 from 2010. Of the 15.1% of women who indicated experiencing unwanted sexual contact, 29% (10 percentage points lower than 2010) indicated they experienced unwanted sexual touching only. Twenty-two percent (unchanged from 2010) indicated the incident included attempted sex, with or without sexual touching; and 43% (13 percentage points higher than 2010) indicated they experienced completed sex, with or without sexual touching and/or attempted sex.

Unwanted Sexual Contact Details. Of the 15.1% of women who indicated experiencing unwanted sexual contact, 100% identified the offender as male (unchanged from 2010), and most (76%—unchanged from 2010) indicated the offender was a fellow midshipman. Sixty-five percent indicated alcohol and/or drugs were involved and 9% indicated threats and physical force were used (both unchanged from 2010). Eleven percent (unchanged from 2010) indicated they reported the incident to a military authority or organization. The main reasons those women chose to report the incident were: to seek closure on the incident (83%), to seek help dealing with an emotional incident (74%), and it was the right thing to do (72%). The main reasons women chose not to report the incident were: they took care of it themselves (77%—10 percentage points higher than 2010), they did not want people gossiping about them (71%—unchanged from 2010), and they did not want anyone to know (68%—7 percentage points higher than 2010).

Prior Unwanted Sexual Contact. Students were asked to indicate if they experienced any of the unwanted sexual contact behaviors prior to entering the Academy. The prior experience rate was 22.3% for women and 3.8% for men.

Unwanted Gender-Related Behaviors. Sixty-one percent of women (unchanged from 2010) and 10% of men (7 percentage points lower than 2010) indicated experiencing sexual harassment in 2012.

Ninety percent of women and 51% of men indicated experiencing crude/offensive behavior (both unchanged from 2010). Sixty-three percent of women and 19% of men indicated experiencing unwanted sexual attention (both unchanged from 2010). Twenty-one percent of women and 5% of men indicated experiencing sexual coercion (both unchanged from 2010). Ninety-four percent of women (2 percentage points lower than 2010) and 46% of men (unchanged from 2010) indicated experiencing sexist behavior.

Unwanted Gender-Related Behavior Details. Ninety-six percent of women and 61% of men indicated experiencing one or more of the unwanted gender-related behaviors (i.e., crude/offensive behavior, unwanted sexual attention, sexual coercion, sexist behavior) in 2012. Of those, the majority of women (81%—unchanged from 2010) and men (70%—6 percentage points higher than 2010) identified the offender as a fellow midshipman. Six percent of women (3 percentage points lower than 2010) and 3% of men (unchanged from 2010) discussed the situation with a military authority or organization.

Stalking. Few women (5.8%—unchanged from 2010) and men (1.0%—unchanged from 2010) indicated that they experienced stalking-related behaviors that caused them fear of physical harm or sexual assault (the requirement to meet the legal definition of stalking).

U.S. Air Force Academy

Unwanted Sexual Contact. Overall, 11.2% of women and 1.7% of men indicated they experienced unwanted sexual contact in 2012. There were no changes in the percentages of women or men in 2012 from 2010. Of the 11.2% of women who indicated experiencing unwanted sexual contact, 19% (unchanged from 2010) indicated they experienced unwanted sexual touching only. Twenty-two percent (11 percentage points lower than 2010) indicated the incident included attempted sex, with or without sexual touching; and 54% (15 percentage points higher than 2010) indicated they experienced completed sex, with or without sexual touching and/or attempted sex.

Unwanted Sexual Contact Details. Of the 11.2% of women who indicated experiencing unwanted sexual contact, nearly all (97%—3 percentage points lower than 2010) identified the offender as male, and most (85%—unchanged from 2010) indicated the offender was a fellow cadet. Sixty percent (12 percentage points higher than 2010) indicated alcohol and/or drugs were involved and 10% (unchanged from 2010) indicated threats and physical force were used. Fifteen percent (unchanged from 2010) indicated they reported the incident to a military authority or organization. The main reasons those women chose to report the incident were: to seek help dealing with an emotional incident (82%), to stop the offender from hurting others (74%), to seek justice (64%), and it was the right thing to do (64%). The main reasons women chose not to report the incident were: they took care of it themselves (66%—unchanged from 2010), they did not want anyone to know (63%—unchanged from 2010), and they did not want people gossiping about them (62%—unchanged from 2010).

Prior Unwanted Sexual Contact. Students were asked to indicate if they experienced any of the unwanted sexual contact behaviors prior to entering the Academy. The prior experience rate was 22.9% for women and 4.6% for men.

Unwanted Gender-Related Behaviors. Forty-four percent of women (9 percentage points lower than 2010) and 11% of men (unchanged from 2010) indicated experiencing sexual harassment in 2012.

Seventy-seven percent of women (7 percentage points lower than 2010) and 43% of men (4 percentage points lower than 2010) indicated experiencing crude/offensive behavior. Fifty-two percent of women (5 percentage points lower than 2010) and 11% of men (unchanged from 2010) indicated experiencing unwanted sexual attention. Seventeen percent of women (3 percentage points lower than 2010) and 3% of men (unchanged from 2010) indicated experiencing sexual coercion. Eighty-five percent of women (4 percentage points lower than 2010) and 37% of men (unchanged from 2010) indicated experiencing sexist behavior.

Unwanted Gender-Related Behavior Details. Eighty-nine percent of women and 51% of men indicated experiencing one or more of the unwanted gender-related behaviors (i.e., crude/offensive behavior, unwanted sexual attention, sexual coercion, sexist behavior) in 2012. Of those, the majority of women (80%) and men (72%) identified the offender as a fellow cadet (both unchanged from 2010). Six percent of women and 0% of men discussed the situation with a military authority or organization (both unchanged from 2010).

Stalking. Few women (4.9%—unchanged from 2010) and men (0.3%—unchanged from 2010) indicated that they experienced stalking-related behaviors that caused them fear of physical harm or sexual assault (the requirement to meet the legal definition of stalking).

U.S. Coast Guard Academy

Unwanted Sexual Contact. Overall, 9.8% of women and 0.7% of men indicated they experienced unwanted sexual contact in 2012. The percentage of women was higher in 2012 than in 2010 and the percentage of men was lower. Of the 9.8% of women who indicated experiencing unwanted sexual contact, 23% (12 percentage points lower than 2010) indicated they experienced unwanted sexual touching only. Thirty-nine percent (22 percentage points higher than 2010) indicated the incident included attempted sex, with or without sexual touching; and 39% (unchanged from 2010) indicated they experienced completed sex, with or without sexual touching and/or attempted sex.

Unwanted Sexual Contact Details. Of the 9.8% of women who indicated experiencing unwanted sexual contact, 100% identified the offender as male (7 percentage points higher than 2010), and most (76%—unchanged from 2010) indicated the offender was a fellow cadet. Fifty-nine percent (unchanged from 2010) indicated alcohol and/or drugs were involved and 8% (8 percentage points higher than 2010) indicated threats and physical force were used. Seven percent (12 percentage points lower than 2010) indicated they reported the incident to a military authority or organization. The main reasons women chose not to report the incident were: they took care of it themselves (86%—15 percentage points higher than 2010), they did not think it was important enough to report (73%—unchanged from 2010), and they did not want people gossiping (69%—unchanged from 2010).

Prior Unwanted Sexual Contact. Students were asked to indicate if they experienced any of the unwanted sexual contact behaviors prior to entering the Academy. The prior experience rate was 15.8% for women and 3.0% for men.

Unwanted Gender-Related Behaviors. Forty percent of women (unchanged from 2010) and 10% of men (7 percentage points lower than 2010) indicated experiencing sexual harassment in 2012.

Seventy-six percent of women (unchanged from 2010) and 46% of men (13 percentage points lower than 2010) indicated experiencing crude/offensive behavior. Forty-two percent of women (6 percentage points higher than 2010) and 13% of men (7 percentage points lower than 2010) indicated experiencing unwanted sexual attention. Eleven percent of women (unchanged from 2010) and 4% of men (2 percentage points lower than 2010) indicated experiencing sexual coercion. Seventy-seven percent of women (3 percentage points lower than 2010) and 40% of men (9 percentage points lower than 2010) indicated experiencing sexist behavior.

Unwanted Gender-Related Behavior Details. Eighty-four percent of women and 55% of men indicated experiencing one or more of the unwanted gender-related behaviors (i.e., crude/offensive behavior, unwanted sexual attention, sexual coercion, sexist behavior) in 2012. Of those, the majority of women (80%—unchanged from 2010) and men (59%—8 percentage points lower than 2010) identified the offender as a fellow cadet. Seven percent of women (3 percentage points higher than 2010) and 2% of men (unchanged from 2010) discussed the situation with a military authority or organization.

Stalking. Few women (3.3%—unchanged from 2010) and men (0.4%—unchanged from 2010) indicated that they experienced stalking-related behaviors that caused them fear of physical harm or sexual assault (the requirement to meet the legal definition of stalking).

NEW VICTIM ADVOCATE PRIVILEGE

ANNEX

Section 1. Part III of the Manual for Courts-Martial, United States, is amended as follows:

    (a) M.R.E. 504 (c)(2)(D) is added to read as follows:

    "(D) Where both parties have been substantial participants in illegal activity, those communications between the spouses during the marriage regarding the illegal activity in which they have jointly participated are not marital communications for purposes of the privilege in subdivision (b) and are not entitled to protection under the privilege in subdivision (b)."

    (b) M.R.E. 513(d)(2) is amended—

        (1) to delete "spouse abuse, child abuse, or" and insert "child abuse or of"; and

        (2) to delete "the person of the other spouse or."

    (c) M.R.E. 514 is added to read as follows:

"Rule 514. Victim advocate–victim privilege

    (a) *General rule of privilege.* A victim has a privilege to refuse to disclose and to prevent any other person from disclosing a confidential communication made between the victim and a victim advocate, in a case arising under the UCMJ, if such communica-

tion was made for the purpose of facilitating advice or supportive assistance to the victim.

(b) *Definitions.* As used in this rule of evidence:

(1) A "victim" is any person who suffered direct physical or emotional
harm as the result of a sexual or violent offense.

(2) A "victim advocate" is a person who is:

(A) designated in writing as a victim advocate;

(B) authorized to perform victim advocate duties in accordance
with service regulations, and is acting in the performance of
those duties; or

(C) certified as a victim advocate pursuant to Federal or State requirements.

(3) A communication is "confidential" if made to a victim advocate
acting in the capacity of a victim advocate and if not intended to be
disclosed to third persons other than:

(A) those to whom disclosure is made in furtherance of the rendi-
tion of advice or assistance to the victim or

(B) an assistant to a victim advocate reasonably necessary for such
transmission of the communication.

(4) An "assistant to a victim advocate" is a person directed by or assigned to assist a victim advocate in providing victim advocate services, or is reasonably believed by the victim to be such.

(5) "Evidence of a victim's records or communications" is testimony of
a victim advocate, or records that pertain to communications by a
victim to a victim advocate, for the purposes of advising or providing supportive assistance to the victim.

(c) *Who may claim the privilege.* The privilege may be claimed by the
victim or any guardian or conservator of the victim. A person
who may claim the privilege may authorize trial counsel or a
defense counsel representing the victim to claim the privilege on
his or her behalf. The victim advocate who received the communication may claim the privilege on behalf of the victim. The
authority of such a victim advocate, guardian, conservator, or a
defense counsel representing the victim to so assert the privilege
is presumed in the absence of evidence to the contrary.

(d) *Exceptions.* There is no privilege under this rule:

(1) when the victim is dead;

(2) when Federal law, State law, or service regulation imposes a
duty to report information contained in a communication;

(3) if the communication clearly contemplated the future commission of a fraud or crime or if the services of the victim
advocate are sought or obtained to enable or aid anyone to
commit or plan to commit what the victim knew or reasonably should have known to be a crime or fraud;

(4) when necessary to ensure the safety and security of military
personnel, military dependents, military property, classified
information, or the accomplishment of a military mission;

(5) when necessary to ensure the safety of any other person
(including the victim) when a victim advocate believes that
a victim's mental or emotional condition makes the victim
a danger; or

(6) when admission or disclosure of a communication is consti-
tutionally required.

(e) *Procedure to determine admissibility of victim records or communications.*

(1) In any case in which the production or admission of records or communications of a victim is a matter in dispute, a party may seek an
interlocutory ruling by the military judge. In order to obtain such a
ruling, the party shall:

(A) file a written motion at least 5 days prior to entry of pleas
specifically describing the evidence and stating the purpose for
which it is sought or offered, or objected to, unless the military
judge, for good cause shown, requires a different time for filing
or permits filing during trial; and

(B) serve the motion on the opposing party, the military judge
and, if practical, notify the victim or the victim's guardian,
conservator, or representative that the motion has been filed
and that the victim has an opportunity to be heard as set forth
in subparagraph (e)(2).

(2) Before ordering the production or admission of evidence of a victim's records or communication, the military judge shall conduct a
hearing. Upon the motion of counsel for either party and upon good
cause shown, the military judge may order the hearing closed. At
the hearing, the parties may call witnesses, including the victim, and
offer other relevant evidence. The victim shall be afforded a reasonable opportunity to attend the hearing and be heard at the victim's
own expense unless the victim has been otherwise subpoenaed or
ordered to appear at the hearing. However, the proceedings shall not
be unduly delayed for this purpose. In a case before a court-martial
composed of a military judge and members, the military judge shall
conduct the hearing outside the presence of the members.

(3) The military judge shall examine the evidence or a proffer thereof *in camera*, if such examination is necessary to rule on the motion.

(4) To prevent unnecessary disclosure of evidence of a victim's records or communications, the military judge may issue protective orders or may admit only portions of the evidence.

(5) The motion, related papers, and the record of the hearing shall be sealed and shall remain under seal unless the military judge or an appellate court orders otherwise.

(d) The following amendments conform M.R.E. 609 to F.R.E. 609:

(1) M.R.E. 609(a) is amended to substitute the words "character for truthfulness" for the word "credibility."

(2) M.R.E. 609(a)(2) is amended to substitute the words "regardless of the punishment, if it readily can be determined that establishing the elements of the crime required proof or admission of an act of dishonesty or false statement by the witness" for the words "if it involved dishonesty or false statement, regardless of the punishment."

(3) M.R.E. 609(c) is amended to substitute the words "a subsequent crime that was punishable by death, dishonorable discharge, or imprisonment in excess of one year" for the words "a subsequent crime which was punishable by death, dishonorable discharge, or imprisonment in excess of one year."

Sec. 2. Part IV of the Manual for Courts-Martial, United States, is amended as follows:

(a) Paragraph 13, Article 89, Disrespect toward a superior commissioned officer, paragraph c.(1) is amended to substitute the words "uniformed service" for "armed forces" and "armed force" everywhere the words "armed forces" or "armed force" appear in that paragraph. (This change is made to clarify that the uniformed officers of the Public Health Service and the National Oceanic and Atmospheric Administration, when assigned to and serving with the armed forces, are included in the definition of a superior commissioned officer.)

(b) Paragraph 35, Article 111, Drunken or reckless operation of vehicle, aircraft or vessel, paragraph f. is amended to read as follows:

"f. *Sample Specification.*

In that _____ (personal jurisdiction data), did (at/ on board _____ location) (subject matter jurisdiction data, if required), on or about _____, 20____, (in the motor pool area) (near the Officer's Club) (at the intersection of _____ and _____) (while in the Gulf of Mexico) (while in flight over

North America) physically control [a vehicle, to wit: (a truck) (a passenger car) (_____)] [an aircraft, to wit: (an AH-64 helicopter) (an F-14A fighter) (a KC-135 tanker) (_____)] [a vessel, to wit: (the aircraft carrier USS _____) (the Coast Guard Cutter _____) (_____)], [while drunk] [while impaired by _____] [while the alcohol concentration in his (blood or breath) equaled or exceeded the applicable limit under subparagraph (b) of the text of the statute in paragraph 35 as shown by chemical analysis] [in a (reckless) (wanton) manner by (attempting to pass another vehicle on a sharp curve) (by ordering that the aircraft be flown below the authorized altitude)] [and did thereby cause said (vehicle) (aircraft) (vessel) to (strike and) (injure_____)]."

    (c) Paragraph 48, Article 123, Forgery, paragraph c.(4) to add the word "to" after the word "liability" the second time it appears in the fifth sentence.

    (d) Paragraph 68b. is added as follows:

"68b. Article 134 (Child pornography)

a. Text of Statute. See paragraph 60.

b. Elements.

1. *Possessing, receiving, or viewing child pornography.*
    (a) That the accused knowingly and wrongfully possessed, received, or viewed child pornography; and
    (b) That, under the circumstances, the conduct of the accused was to the prejudice of good order and discipline in the armed forces or was of a nature to bring discredit upon the armed forces.
2. *Possessing child pornography with intent to distribute.*
    (a) That the accused knowingly and wrongfully possessed child pornography;
    (b) That the possession was with the intent to distribute; and
    (c) That, under the circumstances, the conduct of the accused was to the prejudice of good order and discipline in the armed forces or was of a nature to bring discredit upon the armed forces.
3. *Distributing child pornography.*
    (a) That the accused knowingly and wrongfully distributed child pornography to another; and

(b) That, under the circumstances, the conduct of the accused was to the prejudice of good order and discipline in the armed forces or was of a nature to bring discredit upon the armed forces.

4. *Producing child pornography.*

(a) That the accused knowingly and wrongfully produced child pornography; and

(b) That, under the circumstances, the conduct of the accused was to the prejudice of good order and discipline in the armed forces or was of a nature to bring discredit upon the armed forces.

c. *Explanation.*

(1) "Child Pornography" means material that contains either an obscene visual depiction of a minor engaging in sexually explicit conduct or a visual depiction of an actual minor engaging in sexually explicit conduct.

(2) An accused may not be convicted of possessing, receiving, viewing, distributing, or producing child pornography if he was not aware that the images were of minors, or what appeared to be minors, engaged in sexually explicit conduct. Awareness may be inferred from circumstantial evidence such as the name of a computer file or folder, the name of the host website from which a visual depiction was viewed or received, search terms used, and the number of images possessed.

(3) "Distributing" means delivering to the actual or constructive possession of another.

(4) "Minor" means any person under the age of 18 years.

(5) "Possessing" means exercising control of something. Possession may be direct physical custody like holding an item in one's hand, or it may be constructive, as in the case of a person who hides something in a locker or a car to which that person may return to retrieve it. Possession must be knowing and conscious. Possession inherently includes the power or authority to preclude control by others. It is possible for more than one person to possess an item simultaneously, as when several people share control over an item.

(6) "Producing" means creating or manufacturing. As used in this paragraph, it refers to making child pornography that did not previously exist. It does not include reproducing or copying.

(7) "Sexually explicit conduct" means actual or simulated:

    (a) sexual intercourse or sodomy, including genital-genital, oral-genital, anal-genital, or oral-anal, whether between persons of the same or opposite sex;

    (b) bestiality;

    (c) masturbation;

    (d) sadistic or masochistic abuse; or

    (e) lascivious exhibition of the genitals or pubic area of any person.

(8) "Visual depiction" includes any developed or undeveloped photograph, picture, film or video; any digital or computer image, picture, film, or video made by any means, including those transmitted by any means including streaming media, even if not stored in a permanent format; or any digital or electronic data capable of conversion into a visual image.

(9) "Wrongfulness." Any facts or circumstances that show that a visual depiction of child pornography was unintentionally or inadvertently acquired are relevant to wrongfulness, including, but not limited to, the method by which the visual depiction was acquired, the length of time the visual depiction was maintained, and whether the visual depiction was promptly, and in good faith, destroyed or reported to law enforcement.

(10) On motion of the government, in any prosecution under this paragraph, except for good cause shown, the name, address, social security number, or other nonphysical identifying information, other than the age or approximate age, of any minor who is depicted in any child pornography or visual depiction or copy thereof shall not be admissible and may be redacted from any otherwise admissible evidence, and the panel shall be instructed, upon request of the Government, that it can draw no inference from the absence of such evidence.

d. *Lesser included offenses.*

  (1) *Possessing, receiving, or viewing child pornography.*

  Article 80-attempts.

  (2) *Possessing child pornography with intent to distribute.*

  Article 80-attempts.

  Article 134-possessing child pornography.

  (3) *Distributing child pornography.*

  Article 80-attempts.

  Article 134-possessing child pornography.

  Article 134-possessing child pornography with intent to distribute.

(4) *Producing child pornography.*

Article 80–attempts.

Article 134–possessing child pornography.

e. *Maximum punishment.*

(1) *Possessing, receiving, or viewing child pornography.* Dishonorable discharge, forfeiture of all pay and allowances, and confinement for 10 years.

(2) *Possessing child pornography with intent to distribute.* Dishonorable discharge, forfeiture of all pay and allowances, and confinement for 15 years.

(3) *Distributing child pornography.* Dishonorable discharge, forfeiture of all pay and allowances, and confinement for 20 years.

(4) *Producing child pornography.* Dishonorable discharge, forfeiture of all pay and allowances, and confinement for 30 years.

f. *Sample specification.*

Possessing, receiving, viewing, possessing with intent to distribute, distributing, or producing child pornography.

In that (personal jurisdiction data), did (at/on board—location),on or about _____, 20____ knowingly and wrongfully (possess)(receive)(view) (distribute) (produce) child pornography, to wit: a (photograph)(picture)(film) (video) (digital image)(computer image) of a minor, or what appears to be a minor, engaging in sexually explicit conduct(, with intent to distribute the said child pornography), and that said conduct was (to the prejudice of good order and discipline in the armed forces) (or) (and was) (of a nature to bring discredit upon the armed forces)."

ARTICLE 120 UNIFORM CODE OF MILITARY JUSTICE

45.—Rape and sexual assault generally

[Note: This statute applies to offenses committed on or after 28 June 2012.]

a. *Text of statute.*

(a) *Rape.* Any person subject to this chapter who commits a sexual act upon another person by—

(1) using unlawful force against that other person;

(2) using force causing or likely to cause death or grievous bodily harm to any person;

(3) threatening or placing that other person in fear that any person will be subjected to death, grievous bodily harm, or kidnapping;

(4) first rendering that other person unconscious; or

(5) administering to that other person by force or threat of force, or without the knowledge or consent of that person, a drug, intoxicant, or other similar substance and thereby substantially impairing the ability of that other person to appraise or control conduct; is guilty of rape and shall be punished as a court martial may direct.

(b) *Sexual Assault*. Any person subject to this chapter who—

(1) commits a sexual act upon another person by—
  (A) threatening or placing that other person in fear;
  (B) causing bodily harm to that other person;
  (C) making a fraudulent representation that the sexual act serves a professional purpose; or
  (D) inducing a belief by any artifice, pretense, or concealment that the person is another person;

(2) commits a sexual act upon another person when the person knows or reasonably should know that the other person is asleep, unconscious, or otherwise unaware that the sexual act is occurring; or

(3) commits a sexual act upon another person when the other person is incapable of consenting to the sexual act due to—
  (A) impairment by any drug, intoxicant, or other similar substance, and that condition is known or reasonably should be known by the person; or
  (B) a mental disease or defect, or physical disability, and that condition is known or reasonably should be known by the person; is guilty of sexual assault and shall be punished as a court-martial may direct.

(c) *Aggravated sexual Contact*. Any person subject to this chapter who commits or causes sexual contact upon or by another person, if to do so would violate subsection (a) (rape) had the sexual contact been a sexual act, is guilty of aggravated sexual contact and shall be punished as a court-martial may direct.

(d) *Abusive Sexual Contact*. Any person subject to this chapter who commits or causes sexual contact upon or by another person, if to do so would violate subsection (b) (sexual assault) had the sexual contact been a sexual act, is guilty of abusive sexual contact and shall be punished as a court-martial may direct.

(e) *Proof of Threat.* In a prosecution under this section, in proving that a person made a threat, it need not be proven that the person actually intended to carry out the threat or had the ability to carry out the threat.

(f) *Defenses.* An accused may raise any applicable defenses available under this chapter or the Rules for Court-Martial. Marriage is not a defense for any conduct in issue in any prosecution under this section.

g. Definitions. In this section:

(1) *Sexual act.* The term 'sexual act' means

    (A) contact between the penis, vulva or anus or mouth, and for purposes of this subparagraph contact involving the penis occurs upon penetration, however slight; or

    (B) the penetration, however slight, of the vulva or anus or mouth of another by any part of the body or by any object with an intent to abuse, humiliate, harass, or degrade any person or to arouse or gratify the sexual desire of any person.

(2) *Sexual contact.* The term 'sexual contact' means—

    (A) touching, or causing another person to touch, either directly or through the clothing, the genitalia, anus, groin, breast, inner thigh, or buttocks of any person, with an intent to abuse, humiliate, or degrade any person; or

    (B) any touching, or causing another person to touch, either directly or through the clothing, any body part of any person, if done with an intent to arouse or gratify the sexual desire of any person. Touching may be accomplished by any part of the body.

(3) *Bodily harm.* The term 'bodily harm' means any offensive touching of another, however slight, including any nonconsensual sexual act or nonconsensual sexual contact.

(4) *Grievous bodily harm.* The term 'grievous bodily harm' means serious bodily injury. It includes fractured or dislocated bones, deep cuts, torn members of the body, serious damage to internal organs, and other severe bodily injuries. It does not include minor injuries such as a black eye or a bloody nose.

(5) *Force.* The term 'force' means—

    (A) the use of a weapon;

    (B) the use of such physical strength or violence as is sufficient to overcome, restrain, or injure a person; or

(C) inflicting physical harm sufficient to coerce or compel submission by the victim.

(6) *Unlawful Force.* The term 'unlawful force' means an act of force done without legal justification or excuse.

(7) *Threatening or placing that other person in fear.* The term 'threatening or placing that other person in fear' means a communication or action that is of sufficient consequence to cause a reasonable fear that non-compliance will result in the victim or another person being subjected to the wrongful action contemplated by the communication or action.

(8) *Consent.*

(A) The term 'consent' means a freely given agreement to the conduct at issue by a competent person. An expression of lack of consent through words or conduct means there is no consent. Lack of verbal or physical resistance or submission resulting from the use of force, threat of force, or placing another person in fear does not constitute consent. A current or previous dating or social or sexual relationship by itself or the manner of dress of the person involved with the accused in the conduct at issue shall not constitute consent.

(B) A sleeping, unconscious, or incompetent person cannot consent. A person cannot consent to force causing or likely to cause death or grievous bodily harm or to being rendered unconscious. A person cannot consent while under threat or fear or under the circumstances described in subparagraph (C) or (D) of subsection (b)(1).

(C) Lack of consent may be inferred based on the circumstances of the offense. All the surrounding circumstances are to be considered in determining whether a person gave consent, or whether a person did not resist or ceased to resist only because of another person's actions.

[Note: The subparagraphs that would normally address elements, explanation, lesser included offenses, maximum punishments, and sample specifications are generated under the President's authority to prescribe rules pursuant to Article 36. At the time of publishing this MCM, the President had not prescribed such rules for this version of Article 120. Practitioners should refer to the appropriate statutory language and, to the extent practicable, use Appendix 28 as a guide.]

45a. Article 120a—Stalking

a. Text of statute.

(a) Any person subject to this section:
  (1) who wrongfully engages in a course of conduct directed at a specific person that would cause a reasonable person to fear death or bodily harm, including sexual assault, to himself or herself or a member of his or her immediate family;
  (2) who has knowledge, or should have knowledge, that the specific person will be placed in reasonable fear of death or bodily harm, including sexual assault, to himself or herself or a member of his or her immediate family; and
  (3) whose acts induce reasonable fear in the specific person of death or bodily harm, including sexual assault, to himself or herself or to a member of his or her immediate family; is guilty of stalking and shall be punished as a court-martial may direct.

(b) In this section:

(1) The term "course of conduct" means:
  (A) a repeated maintenance of visual or physical proximity to a specific person; or
  (B) a repeated conveyance of verbal threat, written threats, or threats implied by conduct, or a combination of such threats, directed at or towards a specific person.
    (2) The term "repeated," with respect to conduct, means two or more occasions of such conduct.
    (3) The term "immediate family," in the case of a specific person, means a spouse, parent, child, or sibling of the person, or any other family member, relative, or intimate partner of the person who regularly resides in the household of the person or who within the six months preceding the commencement of the course of conduct regularly resided in the household of the person.

b. Elements.
  (1) That the accused wrongfully engaged in a course of conduct directed at a specific person that would cause a reasonable person to fear

death or bodily harm to himself or herself or a member of his or her immediate family;

(2) That the accused had knowledge, or should have had knowledge, that the specific person would be placed in reasonable fear of death or bodily harm to himself or herself or a member of his or her immediate family; and

(3) That the accused's acts induced reasonable fear in the specific person of death or bodily harm to himself or herself or to a member of his or her immediate family.

c. *Explanation.* See Paragraph 54c(1)(a) for an explanation of "bodily harm".

d. *Lesser included offenses.* Article 80–attempts.

e. *Maximum punishment.* Dishonorable discharge, forfeiture of all pay and allowances, and confinement for 3 years.

51. ARTICLE 125—SODOMY

a. Text of statute.

(a) Any person subject to this chapter who engages in unnatural carnal copulation with another person of the same or opposite sex or with an animal is guilty of sodomy. Penetration, however slight, is sufficient to complete the offense.

(b) Any person found guilty of sodomy shall by punished as a court-martial may direct.

b. Elements.

(1) That the accused engaged in unnatural carnal copulation with a certain other person or with an animal. [Note: Add any of the following as applicable]

(2) That the act was done with a child under the age of 12.

(3) That the act was done with a child who had attained the age of 12 but was under the age of 16.

(4) That the act was done by force and without the consent of the other person.

c. Explanation. It is unnatural carnal copulation for a person to take into that person's mouth or anus the sexual organ of another person or of an animal; or to place that person's sexual organ in the mouth or anus of another person or of an animal; or to have carnal copulation in any opening of the body, except the sexual parts, with another person; or to have carnal copulation with an animal.

d. Lesser included offenses.
   1. With a child under the age of 16.
      (a) Article 125-forcible sodomy (and offenses included therein; see subparagraph (2) below)
      (b) Article 80-attempts
   2. Forcible sodomy.
      (a) Article 125-sodomy (and offences included therein; see subparagraph 3 below)
      (b) Article 134-assault with intent to commit sodomy
      (c) Article 80-attempts.
   3. *Sodomy.* Article 80-attempts
   [Note: Consider lesser included offenses under Art. 120, depending on the factual circumstances in each case.]
e. Maximum punishment.
   (1) *By force and without consent.* Dishonorable discharge, forfeiture of all pay and allowances, and confinement for life without eligibility for parole.
   (2) *With a child who, at the time of the offense, has attained the age of 12 but is under the age of 16 years.* Dishonorable discharge, forfeiture of all pay and allowances, and confinement for 20 years.
   (3) *With a child under the age of 12 years at the time of the offense.* Dishonorable discharge, forfeiture of all pay and allowances, and confinement for life without eligibility for parole.
   (4) *Other cases.* Dishonorable discharge, forfeiture of all pay and allowances, and confinement for 5 years.
f. *Sample specification.*
   In that (personal jurisdiction data), did, (at/on board—location) (subject-matter jurisdiction data, if required), on or about 20, commit sodomy with, (a child under the age of 12) (a child who had attained the age of 12 but was under the age of 16) (by force and without the consent of the said).

GLOSSARY OF ACRONYMS

1SG	First Sergeant (E–8)
2LT	Second Lieutenant
ACOM	Army Commands
ACS	Army Community Service
ACSIM	Assistant Chief of Staff for Installation Management
AFOSI	Air Force Office of Special Investigations
AIT	Advanced Individual Training
AKO	Army Knowledge Online
ALARACT	All Army Activities message
ALMS	Army Learning Management System
AMEDD	Army Medical Department
AOR	Area of Responsibility
AR	Army Regulation
ARI	U.S. Army Research Institute for the Behavioral and Social Sciences
ARNG	Army National Guard
ASA M&RA	Assistant Secretary of the Army for Manpower and Reserve Affairs
ASCC	Army Service Component Commands
ASI	Additional Skill Identifier
AWOL	Absent Without Leave
BCD	Bad Conduct Discharge
BCT	Basic Combat Training
BOLC A	Basic Officer Leader Course—Accession (ROTC)
BOLC B	Basic Officer Leader Course—Branch
BOSS	Better Opportunities for Single Soldiers Program
CAI	Combat Areas of Interest
CCTP	Command Compliance and Training Program

CENTCOM	U.S. Central Command
CES	Civilian Education System
CID	U.S. Army Criminal Investigation Command
COL	Colonel (O-6
CONUS	Continental United States
COPS MPRS	Centralized Operating Police Suite Military Reporting System
CSM	Command Sergeant Major
CW5	Chief Warrant Officer Five
CY	Calendar Year
DA	Department of the Army
DAC	Department of the Army Civilian
DAIG	Department of the Army Inspector General
DD	Dishonorable Discharge
DEOCS	Defense Equal Opportunity Climate Surveys
DoD	Department of Defense
DoDD	Department of Defense Directive
DoDI	Department of Defense Instruction
DoDIG	Department of Defense Inspector General
DoJ	Department of Justice
DSAID	Defense Sexual Assault Incident Database
DSARC	Deployable Sexual Assault Response Coordinator
DTF- SAMS	Defense Task Force on Sexual Assault in the Military Services
E-1	Enlisted 1 (Private)
E-4	Enlisted 4 (Specialist)
E-7	Enlisted 7 (Master Sergeant, Air Force)
EO	Equal Opportunity
EXORD	Execution Order
FETI	Forensic Experiential Trauma Interview
FG	Field Grade
FOB	Forward Operating Base
FORSCOM	U.S. Army Forces Command
FY	Fiscal Year
GAO	Government Accountability Office
GCM	General Court Martial
GO	General Order
GOMOR	General Officer Memorandum of Reprimand
GTSY.com	Good to See You
HASC	House Armed Services Committee
HQDA	Headquarters, Department of the Army
HQE	Highly Qualified Experts

HRC	Human Resources Command
ICRS	Integrated Case Reporting System
IET	Initial Entry Training
IG	Inspector General
IMCOM	Installation Management Command
ISAF	International Security Assistance Force
IWG	International Working Group
JAG	Judge Advocate General
JAGC	Judge Advocate General Corps
JCS	Joint Chiefs of Staff
LOD	Line of Duty
LOE	Lines of Effort
MAJ	Major
MCIO	Military Criminal Investigation Organization
MEDCOM	U.S. Army Medical Command
MEJA	Military Extraterritorial Jurisdiction Act
MILPER	Military Personnel Message
MOA	Memorandum of Agreement
MOU	Memorandum of Understanding
MPO	Military Protective Order
MTF	Military Treatment Facility
MTT	Mobile Training Teams
MVP	Mentors in Violence Prevention
MWR	Morale Welfare and Recreation
NCIS	Naval Criminal Investigative Service
NCO	Noncommissioned Officer
NCOER	Noncommissioned Officer Evaluation Report
NDAA	National Defense Authorization Act
NJP	Non-judicial Punishment
NOVA	National Organization for Victim Assistance
OCONUS	Outside Continental United States
OCPA	Office of the Chief, Public Affairs
OEF	Operation Enduring Freedom
OER	Officer Evaluation Report
OMPF	Official Military Personnel File
OSD	Office of the Secretary of Defense
OTH	Other Than Honorable (discharge)
OTS	Operational Troops Survey
OTJAG	Office of the Judge Advocate General
PCC	Pre-command Course
PFC	Private First Class (E-3)
PME	Professional Military Education

POSH	Prevention of Sexual Harassment
PTSD	Post-traumatic Stress Disorder
PV2	Private (E-2)
RCM	Rule for Court-martial
RN	Registered Nurse
ROI	Report of Investigation
ROTC	Reserve Officers Training Corps
RR	Restricted Report
SAAM	Sexual Assault Awareness Month
SACC	Sexual Assault Care Coordinators
SACP	Sexual Assault Clinical Providers
SADMS	Sexual Assault Database Management System
SAFE	Sexual Assault Forensic Exam
SAMFE	Sexual Assault Medical Forensic Examiner
SAMM	Sexual Assault Medical Management Conference
SANE	Sexual Assault Nurse Examiner
SAPR	Sexual Assault Prevention and Response Program
SAPRO	Sexual Assault Prevention and Response Program Office
SARB	Sexual Assault Review Board
SARC	Sexual Assault Response Coordinator
SCM	Summary Court-martial
SFC	Sergeant First Class (E-7)
SGT	Sergeant (E-5)
SHARP	Sexual Harassment/Assault Response and Prevention Program
SJA	Staff Judge Advocate
SME	Subject Matter Expert
SOL	Statute of Limitations
SOT	Sex Offender Treatment Group
SPCM	Special Court-martial
SPCMCA	Special Court-martial Convening Authority
SSG	Staff Sergeant (E-6)
SSMP	Sample Survey of Military Personnel
SVP	Special Victims Prosecutor
SVU	Special Victims Unit
SVUIC	Special Victims Unit Instructor Course
TCAP	Trial Counsel Assistance Program
TDY	Temporary Duty
TF	Total Forfeiture
TJAGLCS	The Judge Advocate General's School and Legal Center
TRADOC	U.S. Army Training and Doctrine Command
TSP	Training Support Packages

UCMJ	Uniform Code of Military Justice
UOTHC	Under Other-Than-Honorable Conditions
UR	Unrestricted Report
USACIL	U.S. Army Criminal Investigation Laboratory
USAF	U.S. Air Force
USAFE	U.S. Air Force, Europe
USAMAA	U.S. Army Manpower Analysis Agency
USAMPS	U.S. Army Military Police School
USAREC	U.S. Army Recruiting Command
USAREUR	U.S. Army, Europe
USARPAC	U.S. Army, Pacific
USC	Unwanted Sexual Contact
USDB	U.S. Disciplinary Barracks
USD P&R	Under Secretary of Defense for Personnel and Readiness
USMA	U.S. Military Academy
USMC	U.S. Marine Corps
USN	U.S. Navy
UVA	Unit Victim Advocate
VA	Victim Advocate
VWL	Victim/Witness Liaison
WO1	Warrant Office One
XO	Executive Officer

INDEX

ABOUT THE AUTHORS

Cheryl Lawhorne Scott is a clinical therapist with an 18-year track record of counseling services specializing in trauma care; post-traumatic stress; and traumatic brain injury treatment for wounded, ill, and injured service members and their families. As a senior consultant under the Office of the Secretary of Defense, she is part of a team that seeks innovative and proactive ways to enhance resources and services to military members and their families.

She recently participated in the corporate mission, vision, and implementation of projects for the Department of Defense to align current and future strategic plans and objectives. She possesses proven expertise in both program management and clinical expertise in research, business development, and wounded care. She is proud spouse and teammate to Lieutenant Colonel Jeff Scott, and mom to Evan and Quinn.

Don Philpott is editor of *International Homeland Security Journal* and has been writing, reporting, and broadcasting on international events, trouble spots, and major news stories for almost forty years. For twenty years he was a senior correspondent with Press Association—Reuters, the wire service, and traveled the world on assignments including Northern Ireland, Lebanon, Israel, South Africa, and Asia.

He writes for magazines and newspapers in the United States and Europe and is a regular contributor to radio and television programs on security and other issues. He is the author of more than 140 books on a wide range of subjects and has had more than 5,000 articles printed in publications around the world. His recent books include the Military Life series; *Terror—Is America Safe*; *Workplace Violence Prevention*; and the *Education Facility Security Handbook*, all published by Rowman & Littlefield.

LtCol. Jeff Scott is a 26-year prior enlisted U.S. Marine Corps lieutenant colonel who has held various leadership positions throughout his service, with the most recent being the commanding officer of the world's first operational F-35 Lightning II Joint Strike Fighter squadron. In addition to being the first operational F-35 pilot and first operational F-35 commander, LtCol. Scott has received formal service training on sexual assault prevention and response as part of his leadership training and has mentored many Marines. LtCol. Scott has also served with senior leadership at the Pentagon and holds a B.SC. in Finance from San Jose State University and a master's degree in business administration from Boston University.